# MEDICAL HISTORY FOR STUDENTS

To Owsei Temkin

with deep appreciation

John R Green
October 15, 1968

# MEDICAL HISTORY FOR STUDENTS

*By*

**JOHN R. GREEN, M.D.**

*Chairman, Barrow Neurological Institute*
*St. Joseph's Hospital*
*Phoenix, Arizona*
*Lecturer, Department of Zoology*
*History of Medicine*
*Arizona State University*
*Tempe, Arizona*

CHARLES C THOMAS · PUBLISHER

*Springfield · Illinois · U.S.A.*

*Published and Distributed Throughout the World by*
CHARLES C THOMAS · PUBLISHER
BANNERSTONE HOUSE
301-327 East Lawrence Avenue, Springfield, Illinois, U.S.A.
NATCHEZ PLANTATION HOUSE
735 North Atlantic Boulevard, Fort Lauderdale, Florida, U.S.A.


Library of Congress Catalog Card Number: 68-20785



*Printed in the United States of America*

**K-8**

*This book is affectionately dedicated*
*to my wife and children,*
*Georgia, Charles A. III, and Gretchen*

# Preface

With the encouragement and stimulation of Owsei Temkin, M.D., Professor of History of Medicine at the Johns Hopkins University School of Medicine, the author developed a course of instruction about this subject for undergraduate and graduate students at Arizona State University in 1957. A series of lectures has been offered each year since then and listed in the curriculum as Course B-218—Outlines of the History of Medicine. An elective subject, the classes have been enlarged each year to meet the requests of premedical students and those in a number of other disciplines. In order to supplement notes and slides, a syllabus was prepared in 1961 and now, because of requests by a considerable number of students and medical colleagues, this lecture series and syllabus are being revised into a slightly expanded format—*Medical History for Students*. Our hope is that such a presentation will be rewarding to students, medical colleagues, nurses and all individuals who are interested in medicine. It is recognized that scholars of medical history are deeply involved in specific aspects of these subjects which can only be mentioned or alluded to in this introductory text. A list of references for reading is compiled following the last chapter for those students who wish to continue to expand their understanding of this interesting subject. The author acknowledges his debt to these publications and also to his students and colleagues for the development of this book.

Finally, it is a pleasure to record my thanks to members of the Staff of the Barrow Neurological Institute of St. Joseph's Hospital, particularly (Mrs.) Nancy Maxwell, my efficient secretary, De Block and Mr. Cecil Gilliam, for their illustrations and photography, respectively, Miss Isabelle Anderson for library assistance and also to Charles C Thomas, Publisher for bringing out this edition in such a pleasing format.

J.R.G.

# List of Illustrations

# Contents

# MEDICAL HISTORY FOR STUDENTS

*The history of medicine—can claim a very special interest in the history of the development of human thought, for no other history is better adapted to demonstrate that a correct criticism of the sources of our knowledge is practically one of the most important duties of true philosophy.*
—HERMANN VON HELMHOLTZ

# I Introduction

THE HISTORY of medical thought has been a succession of errors, victories and by no means has it been an ascending road of progress. One quickly learns from this that change and progress are not synonymous. It is essential and fascinating to study medical history in various ways. Human instinct, fear, hope, faith, as well as great political and social events of the day, influence medical thought. New ideas are frequently forgotten and then rediscovered, new facts may lead to important social legislation, and the history of individuals is inseparable from the history of ideas and facts.

Santayana reminds us that "those who cannot remember the past are condemned to repeat it." The noted Viennese surgeon, Billroth, put the same thought in these words, "Only the man who is familiar with the art and science of the past is competent to aid in its progress in the future."

Three other quotations should suffice to emphasize the importance of the force of history on our lives:

By despising all that has preceded us, we teach others to despise ourselves. Where there is no established scale nor rooted faith in excellence, all superiority—our own as well as others—soon comes to the ground.—WILLIAM HAZLITT, *On Reading New Books.*

In the study of some apparently new problems, we often make progress by reading the work of the great men of the past.—DOCTOR CHARLES H. MAYO.

In the continual remembrance of the glorious past, individuals and nations find their noblest inspiration.—SIR WILLIAM OSLER.

The educational value of medical history was sporadically recognized by a few outstanding individuals from civilization to civilization. However, there was almost complete neglect of history by leading medical men and institutions as late as 1889, when Theodore Puschmann, Professor of the History of Medicine at the University of Vienna, discussed this state of affairs in the following manner.

The use of historical studies manifests itself in three ways: First, they complete general education; then, they form the foundation of professional knowledge and fortify it; and finally, they further the education and ennobling of the character.

When the history of medicine and of the sciences is seen as a part of the general history of culture and is thus presented, when the teacher follows its relation to the other arts and sciences, and vice versa, calls attention to the influence of the latter on natural science and medicine, when he considers at once political events and social conditions, and gives to the whole the characteristic aura of the age, his lectures will complement and broaden the students in every way.

In the same year of 1889, the Johns Hopkins Medical History Club was organized because of the stimulation of the new Professor of Medicine, William Osler, and a beginning was made in what has now become a tradition. Although a number of medical schools offer formalized courses of instruction in the history of medicine, only a few universities have such an elective in their curricula of study. We have observed such an elective in operation during the past decade and believe that the efforts of all who are concerned are rewarding. The text which follows is based upon these lectures.

*He who ceases to try to do better ceases to do well.*—Oliver Cromwell

# II Primitive Medicine

Primitive medical concepts and practices began with the first man on earth and have not entirely disappeared today. Man's time began over a million years ago and may be divided into the Paleolithic, Mesolithic and Neolithic primitive periods—the age of archaic medicine (Fig. 1).

Ninety-nine percent of man's time on earth, in excess of one million years, ended in about 8000 B.C. and has been called the *Paleolithic* period. The tragic tale of prehistoric man and his diseases is known to us, in small measure, because of fossils, bones and teeth. The study of the abnormalities found in these remains is known as *paleopathology*. This study includes both man and animals. A hemangioma in a bone of a Mesozoic dinosaur is probably the earliest-known tumor. Fractures, dental caries, parasitic diseases, arthritis, osteomyelitis and actinomycosis have been described.

*Pithecanthropus erectus* is regarded as the oldest-known representative of man on earth. He lived about five hundred thousand years ago in Java and his femur showed an exostosis which possibly represents the oldest example of human pathology. *Cro-Magnon Man* was massive-brained and lived about 25,000 B.C. *Neanderthal Man* lived during the last glacial age and was followed by *Homo sapiens* in about 8000 B.C. These prehistoric men used animal teeth and horns as weapons and probably communicated with their fellow creatures by means of grunts, gestures and blows.

With the discovery of stone implements, such as the flint axe, a stone fingernail, and similar tools, the *Mesolithic* period started in approximately 8000 B.C. We know something of these primitive men because of carved stones, cave paintings, myths and legends and the magical thought of primitive tribes of today among people who are still isolated from the civilization of our time.

The *Neolithic* period began about 4000 B.C. in Europe and Asia. These people developed a food-producing economy as the result of four new inventions: (1) agriculture; (2) domesticated animals; (3) pottery, and (4) polished stone tools.

The medicine of these primitive cultures was of four types: (1) instinctive; (2) empirical; (3) magical, and (4) priestly.

*Instinctive medical practice* was surely the first among primitive peoples. Maternal solicitude is instinctive for the preservation of the race and animals have always treated themselves in this manner. Instinctive attempts at self-healing included licking, sucking and blowing on lesions.

*Empirical medicine* was derived from instinctive ideas but was subordinated to current ideas of causal relation. If the cause was not visible or apparent, distant agents such as the stars or spirits were felt to be the cause. Accordingly, spells, natural forces, plants and other methods of treatment were followed. Thus, when instinctive medical practices became stereotyped, the ritual became as important as the treatment.

*Magical medicine* originated from empirical medicine and was based upon the belief that diseases were caused by supernatural causes. This led to medical mythology, medicine men, masks, beads, tattooing and numerous other interesting devices.

*Priestly medicine* developed from this primitive empirical and magical medicine when religious ideas evolved to satisfy the collective needs of the tribe. Castes were organized in which the practice of magical medicine was conserved as a traditional secret and sanctuaries became the temples and schools of medicine.

Neolothic men who lived in various parts of Europe and Asia were Caucasians, Mongolians and Negroids. They gradually developed social habits and community life, devised a mathematic system based on counting fingers and toes, learned to use the wheel, discovered ceramics, cultivated plants, invented textiles, domesticated animals, polished stones and set the stage for a series of civilizations which were to follow.

Magical medicine still prevails in present-day primitive communities. The medicine man or shaman practiced exorcism and

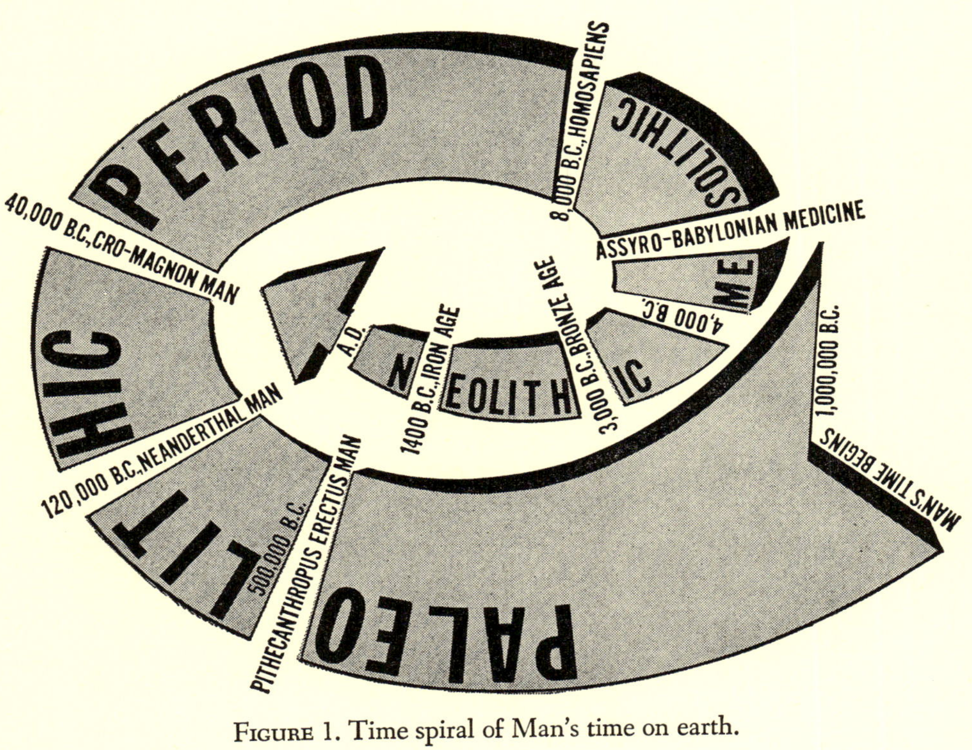


FIGURE 1. Time spiral of Man's time on earth.

was usually the most brilliant man in his community, combining the functions of doctor, magician, priest, statesman and troubadour.

Surgery of the primitive peoples possessed an astonishing degree of technical efficiency. The most ancient instruments were but sharpened stones. Trephining of the skull was carried out among many Neolithic peoples to remove splinters and fragments of the fractured skull, for magical purposes to release evil spirits, and was also done on the dead who had previously been trephined, in order to remove amulets (Fig. 2). These were sometimes strung as necklaces to protect the living from the fate of the deceased. Many of these patients survived the surgery of trephination of the skull. The evidence of this is the finding of healed bone-edges around the openings made in skulls which had been trephined during this period and found much later. This operation is probably the earliest of which we have tangible evidence (Fig. 3).

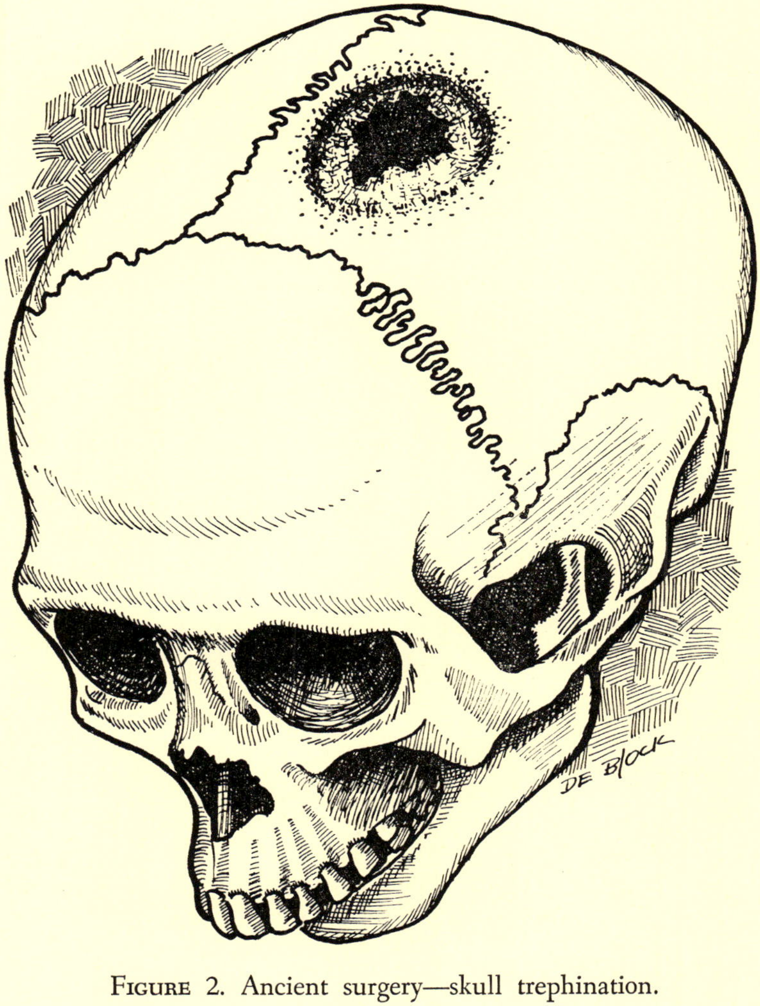


FIGURE 2. Ancient surgery—skull trephination.

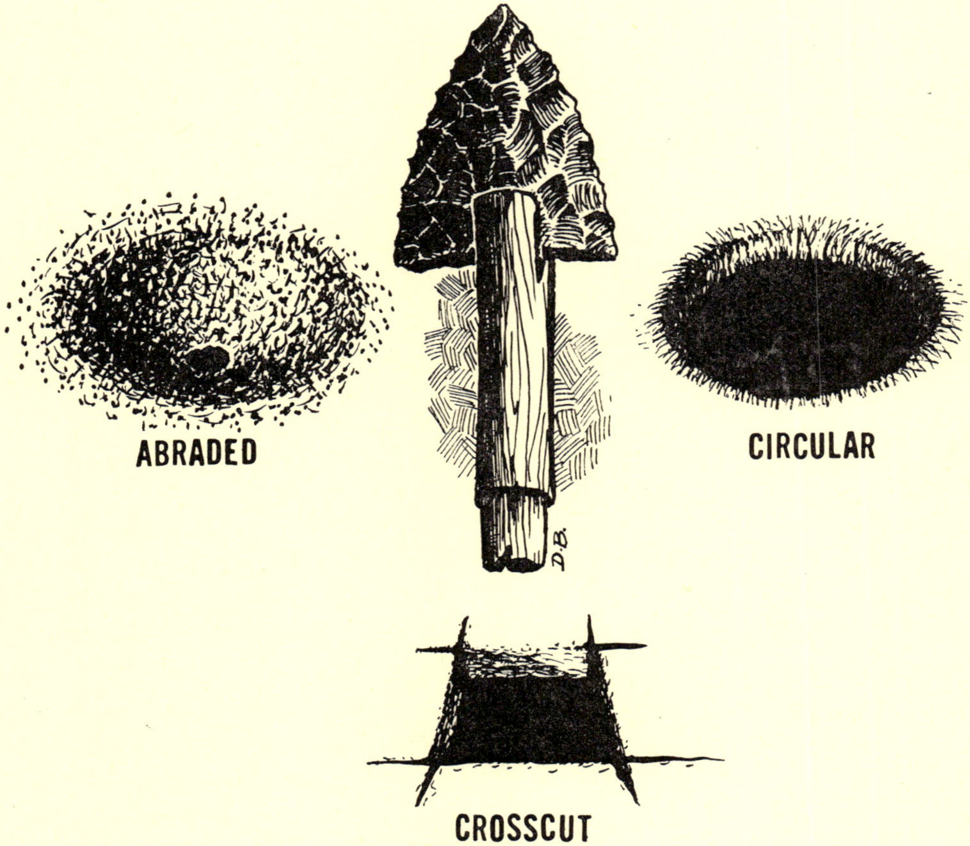

FIGURE 3. Stone trephine and methods of trephination.

The *Bronze Age* began in the Near East in about 3000 B.C. and the *Iron Age* began in Asia Minor about 1400 B.C. Knives, saws, files and other instruments of these metals were developed for surgical procedures and used by the primitive surgeons. It is known that amputations were done during the neolithic period. Mutilating operations to the genital organs, such as castration and circumcision, were done during this period on the basis of magical concepts and to replace human sacrifice.

Thus, mystic faith and empiric experience, based upon seeing and believing, were the first attitudes adopted by the primitive physician. The rational knowledge of disease was destined to evolve with the development of civilizations.

*History is philosophy teaching by example and also by warning. Its two eyes are geography and chronology.*—DIONYSIUS

# III Assyro-Babylonian Medicine

THE FIRST KNOWN civilization was located on a plain, between the Euphrates and Tigris Rivers, on the eastern basin of the Mediterranean Sea (Fig. 4). This began around the fourth and fifth millennia before Christ, and by 4000 B.C., these people had developed a systematic medical concept from which was derived Assyro-Babylonian medicine. These food-producing peoples, whose food-gathering forebears had lived in caves in the northern uplands, slowly settled the valleys and plains between these great rivers and as far to the south as the Persian Gulf. They built and rebuilt villages, created special dwellings for their offerings and sacrifices to benevolent gods, grew crops, raised herds and eventually created towns and cities. These people were the Sumerians.

The Sumerians thought of their gods as human in form, thought and action and created imposing temples in each city as monuments to the power of the principal gods in whom all wealth was vested. The priestly caste tended the vast holdings of the temples, worked their land with the help of farmers on a sharecropping basis, and created the world's oldest written records on clay cylinder seals. The Sumerians created the Ziggurat, the famed Biblical Tower of Babel at Uruk.

The tradition of kingship began in the early days of the Sumerian city-state organization. Although the leader was initially chosen by an assembly of free citizens, he eventually became a hereditary ruler and his palace rivaled the religious temple in wealth and power. The excavations of the royal tombs at Ur revealed such wealth and power. The early written language of the Sumerians was a pictographic script of about nine hundred signs. These were gradually modified into a linear script by the introduction of marks which were meant to clarify ideographic and phonetic values. The Sumerians continued the practice of magical and priestly medicine and knew almost nothing of astronomy.

The Akkadians gained control of all Mesopotamia, by force of arms, by breaking the power of the Sumerians in about 2500 B.C. The Akkadians were a Semitic people and their leader became known in history as Sargon who founded Akkad as his capitol. Barbarian invaders, the Guti, conquered the Akkadians in the twenty-third century B.C. and ruled for about a century. Sumerian dominion was then reestablished and centered in Ur and La-

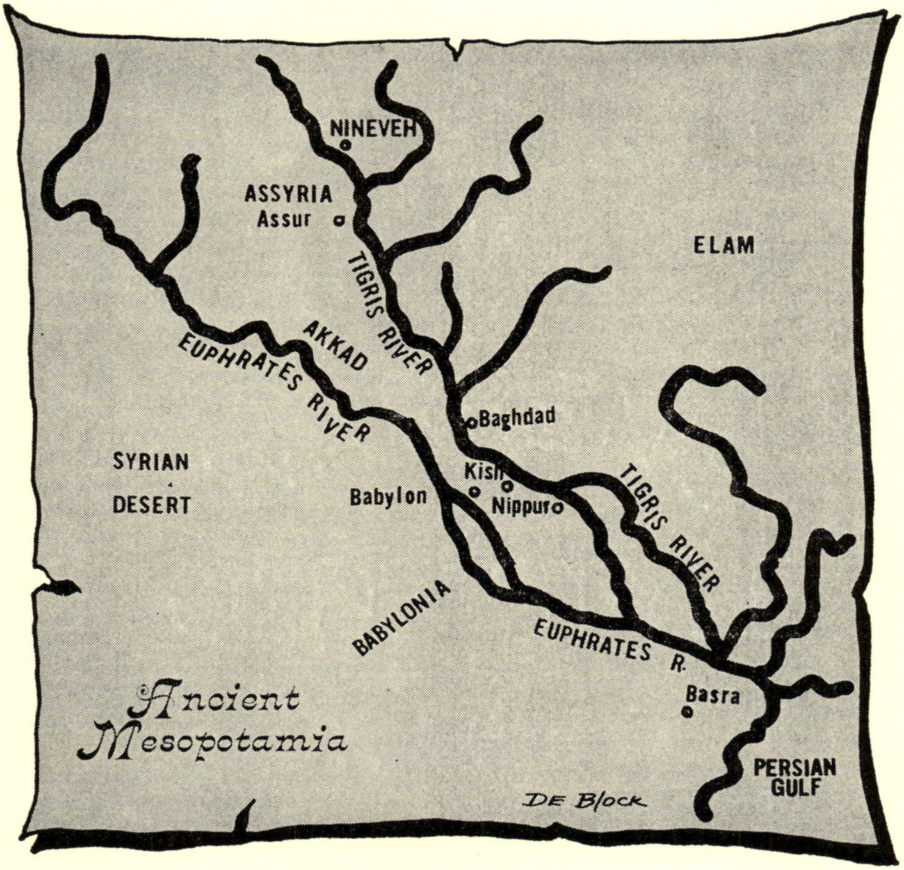


FIGURE 4.

gash. The Sumerian regime collapsed at Ur in 2015 B.C. under the combined attacks by the Elamites from the east and by the Semites from the west. The Semites established their hegemony through local rulers in a number of cities.

The first dynasty of Babylon was established in about 1900 B.C. and the sixth king of this dynasty was Hammurabi (1792–1750 B.C.).

The Babylonians inherited from the Sumerians their customs, laws, and doctrines and it is to them that we owe the great development of science and art. Babylon became the home of famous schools and temples and this area represented the center of Mediterranean civilization during the second millennium. The government was a powerful monarchy. Medicine was entirely in the hands of the priestly caste and the surgeon was the slave of the physician.

The study of astronomy led to an expression of medical principles. The sun was considered to be the first source of fertility and the origin of every form of life. The people considered water to be the source of fertility of the soil, necessary for life and beneficient, but also to have threatening and devastating possibilities. They considered definite relationships between the movement of stars and the seasons with the manifestations of certain diseases.

Four interesting concepts developed during this period, namely: (1) metamorphosis (a relationship and union of man, animals and plants); (2) reincarnation (resurrection in another form of life); (3) astrology (the destiny of man being determined by the stars), and (4) that birth anomalies represented an evil omen.

Blood was considered to be the carrier of every vital function and the liver was considered to be the essential organ to every life process because it was observed to receive all of the blood from the body. This concept led to the practice of liver divination which took several forms. This organ was examined first of all in sacrificial animals to derive divinations and auspices from its forms, position and any irregularities that it might possess. The priestly physician would mark out areas of the liver in relation to the position of the stars and divine from this technique the destiny of the individual. The sick child would be requested to breathe into the nostrils of a sheep and the sheep would then be sacrificed so that its liver could be examined for this purpose. This practice was very common and was transmitted later by the Hittites to the Etruscans in Italy.

Medical writings of the day described fevers, apoplexy, phthisis, plague, eye, ear, nose and throat diseases, rheumatism, tumors, abscesses, diseases of the heart and skin, venereal diseases and many others. Toothache was thought to be due to the gnawing of a worm, a belief that persisted for centuries.

Hammurabi, who was the sixth king of the first dynasty of Babylon, for the first time established the concept of the responsibility of the physician. This regards the physician strictly as a professional, describes something of the frequency of surgical procedures and the penalties for morbidity and mortality. According to the *Code of Hammurabi* (Fig. 5), if a slave patient died as a result of treatment by a physician,

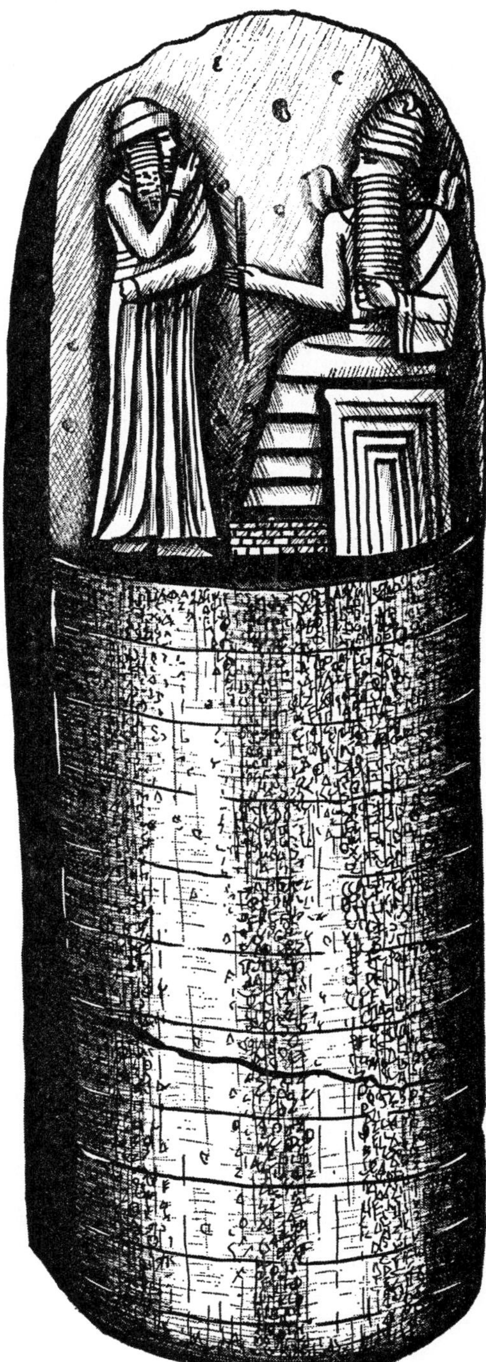

FIGURE 5. Code of Hammurabi of Babylon.

the physician had to replace the slave. If the slave patient lost an eye, the physician had to pay half of the value of the slave to his owner. The surgeon's hands were cut off entirely in the event that a free patient lost his life as a result of an operation. This same *Code* indicates with particular exactness the diseases which could annul or invalidate a lay contract regarding the purchase of a slave. Two of these diseases were cited under the names of "Bennu" and "Siptu," which have been identified by some as epilepsy and leprosy, respectively.

Hammurabi's successors in Babylonia gradually lost power. The state of Assyria became independent, expanded and then became dominant in Mesopotamia. The Assyrians had started as one of the Sumerian satellites in a small city-state built around Ashur in the middle of the Tigris as early as the second millennium. Their kings built vast monuments with the labor of subjugated peoples. The triumphs of King Ashurbanipal were celebrated by the building of his capital at Nineveh. His palace was richly ornamented and contained a great library. The remains of this library, twenty-five thousand tablets, constitute one of the chief sources of our knowledge of Babylonian medicine.

Nineveh was captured in 612 B.C. by the king of Babylon. His son, Nebuchadnezzar, rebuilt the capital and made it the last great center of Mesopotamian culture.

Meanwhile, during the seventh century B.C., a small Persian kingdom grew into an empire and under Darius (521–485 B.C.) conquered the territory from the Nile to India. Persian culture synthesized the heritage of nomadic peoples with that of the most highly developed civilizations of the ancient world. The Persians were, in turn, overcome by Alexander the Great in the fourth century B.C.

## SUMMARY

The Assyro-Babylonian civilization witnessed the slow evolution of demonic medicine into priestly and lay medicine, with a persistent retention of empirical medicine. These were the first people who concerned themselves with human anatomy as well as with that of animals, and who first codified the responsibility of the physician.

*Egypt is the gift of the Nile.*—HERODOTUS

# IV Egyptian Medicine

THE ANCIENT CIVILIZATION of the Egyptians in the Valley of the Nile River developed parallel to and perhaps independently of the great civilization in Mesopotamia. The Nile runs for about seven hundred miles from the first cataract at Aswan to the delta. The valley itself is narrow and is sealed off from the desert by towering rock cliffs.

The early Egyptians, whose ancestors had probably roamed North Africa, gradually developed Neolithic settlements in about 5000 B.C. and established the First Dynasty nearly 2,000 years later under Menes.

Lower Egypt was the marshland of the delta region and Upper Egypt began with the first cataract and extended southward where canal and reservoir construction was developed (Fig. 6). Menes ruled over a united Egypt and was responsible for the earliest damming of the Nile. The Egyptians believed that the control of the flood waters could not have been accomplished without divine guidance under the leadership of the king. They worshipped numerous gods, especially the sun, and considered that safeguarding the existence of the king for eternity was a sacred obligation. The Egyptians also believed that the preservation of physical aspects of life on earth was essential for life in the hereafter. This concept was the basis of tombs and mummification.

The Old Kingdom was initiated by the Pharaoh Zoser during the Third Dynasty about 2700 B.C. His counselor was Imhotep, a master of medicine and a brilliant architect. Zoser's creation of a dwelling worthy of his immortal spirit engaged the resources of the entire land. The world's first large-scale stone building, the gleaming limestone Step pyramid, nearly 200 feet high, was created by Imhotep for Zoser at Saqqarah near Memphis. Imhotep's workmen used only small stone blocks but the great tradition of monumental tomb building led to techniques in which more than two million stone blocks, weighing from two to fifteen tons, were used in the pyramids of later dynasties. The great Sphinx at Giza appears as a mythical image of the pharaoh with the body of a lion, meant to symbolize his power. This sphinx is usually regarded as the work of Khafre of the Fourth Dynasty.

The Middle Kingdom developed in southern Egypt as a new confederation around 2100 B.C. Thebes was its capital and its monarch was Intef. The classical age of Egyptian literature began during this period. It was no longer purely religious and fiction began with the story of Sinuhet. Architecture and the plastic arts

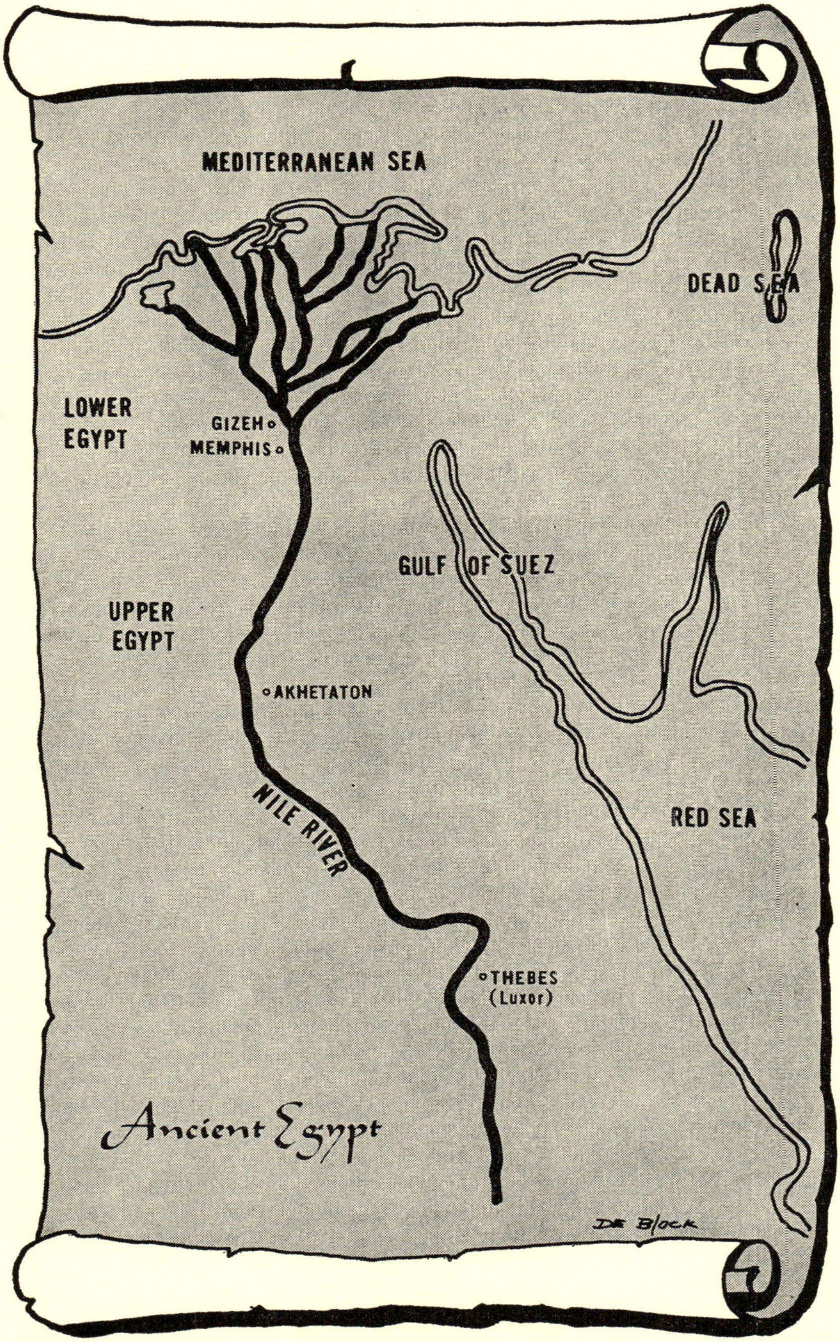
MEDITERRANEAN SEA
DEAD SEA
LOWER EGYPT
GIZEH
MEMPHIS
GULF OF SUEZ
UPPER EGYPT
AKHETATON
NILE RIVER
RED SEA
THEBES (Luxor)
Ancient Egypt
DE BLOCK

FIGURE 6.

flourished. The powers of provincial barons were curbed and wars of conquest were begun. Mining operations and hydraulic works were developed. The Hyksos dominated the Middle Kingdom rulers in 1720 B.C. The Hyksos were a mixture of Semites and Hurrins from Palestine, Syria and farther north and brought the horse into Egypt.

The New Empire began in 1567 B.C. Egypt became an imperial military power engaged in campaigns of conquest and expelled the Hyksos. Tributes and alliances were obtained from the south and from the east to the Red Sea. Thebes remained the capital city for over 600 years. The Pharaoh Ikhnaton (1375–1358 B.C.) envisioned a single God for the whole world (Aton, the sun disk) but his religious reformation did not survive him.

The unsettled and variegated political history of Egypt affected the development of its medical culture over a period of five or six thousand years. Thus, it was predominately mystical and priestly in those times in which the oriental influence prevailed, and empirical and realistic in those places where contact with nature persisted the longest.

Egyptian mythology changed with the times and places and emphasized the concern of the gods with health. Thoth was the most important god of health, allegedly revealing the healing art to Egypt. The well-known insignia for prescriptions, Rx, originated with a legend from this period. It was said that Horus, the son of Isis, lost his vision after a vicious attack by Seth, the demon of evil. Isis called upon Thoth who promptly restored the eye and its powers. The eye of Horus became the Egyptian symbol of godly protection and recovery and is written today on every prescription as Rx.

Imhotep (pronounced I-em-hetep) was active as grand vizier, architect, priest, scribe, sage, astronomer and magician-physician (Fig. 7). His name signifies "He who cometh in peace." He initiated a medical cult as early as 2750 B.C. and preceded Aesculapius by many centuries. In addition to planning and supervising the world's first large-scale stone building (Zoser's pyramid at Saqqarah) Imhotep must have been an outstanding physician and teacher because he was worshipped as a medical demagogue within a few centuries after his death, and became a full deity in 525 B.C., when Egypt became a Persian province. The concepts and practices of Imhotep and his followers were duly recorded on papyri and stored. One of these papyri is actually the most important and complete treatise on surgery of all antiquity and was discovered at Luxor by Edwin Smith in 1862. It was believed to have been written about 1700 B.C. as a summation of the knowledge of Imhotep and his disciples. This evidently was a copy of ancient manuscripts written two-hundred or more years previously. These writings outline proper diagnosis, prognosis and treatment in a series of surgical cases. Paralysis of the bladder and intestines is noted in lesions of the spinal cord. The brain is mentioned for the first time in history. Professor J. H. Breasted of the University of Chicago published in facsimile and hieroglyphic transliteration, a translation and commentary on the Edwin Smith Surgical Papyrus. The medical aspects of Egyptian practice were emphasized in another papyrus. This work, known as the Ebers Papyrus, was believed to have been written between

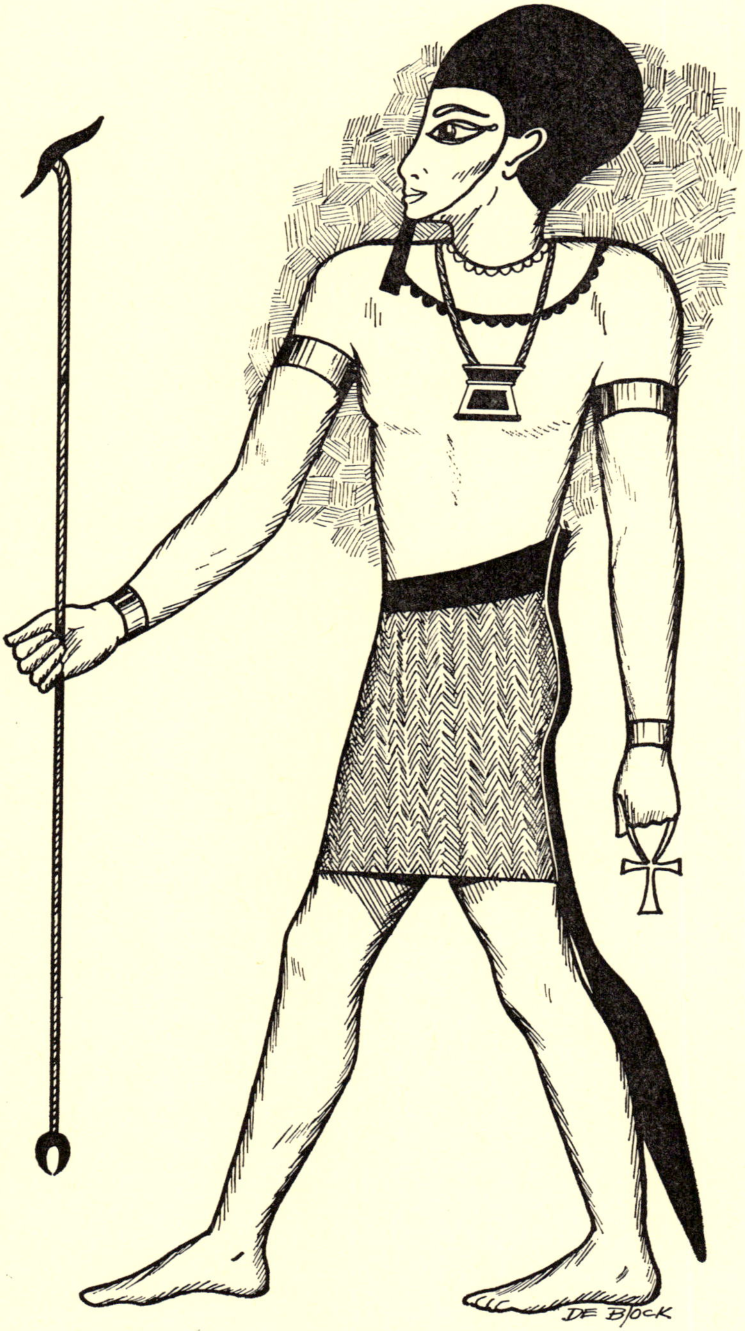


FIGURE 7. Imhotep ("He who cometh in peace").

1553 and 1550 B.C. in one of Imhotep's sanctuaries. Breasted has commented that if the works of Imhotep and his followers had been known as long as those of Hippocrates and his disciples, the title "Father of Medicine" might properly have been considered for Imhotep. In any event, the Edwin Smith and Ebers Papyri are now considered to be among the outstanding writings in medical history.

The anatomical knowledge of the Egyptians was probably less superficial than appears from the study of documents. Mummification during thousands of years, and frequent dissection of animals for religious purposes, must have offered some foundation for knowledge of anatomy. The Ebers Papyrus indicates that the heart was recognized as the center of the blood supply and that "there are vessels attached to it for every member of the body." It also mentions that the motion of the heart can be detected by placing the fingers on the head, the hands, the arms and the legs. The surgeons knew where the major blood vessels were located. In that the hieroglyphics showed the uterus to be bicornate, the heart like that of a cow and the throat the windpipe of cattle, it is apparent that most anatomical knowledge was obtained from animals rather than from man.

Respiration was considered to be the carrier of every vital function and the pneumatic concept was characteristic of Egyptian medicine. The Egyptians noted that cessation of respiration preceded the failure of blood and so blood was considered to be less important than respiration.

Parasites were blamed as the cause for most diseases. Medical problems caused by worms, insects and scorpions were well known. Boils, carbuncles, diseases of the eyes and skin, mastoid disease, alopecia, various fevers and rheumatoid conditions were treated. Dysmenorrhea, prolapse of the uterus and vaginal disease, as well as scanty lactation were mentioned. Syphilis was not recognized.

Physical examination included inspection, palpation and auscultation. The Egyptian physician knew of the examination of the pulse. He was acquainted with listening to the heart and chest and abdomen, according to the Ebers Papyrus ("Here the ear hears beneath").

Therapeutics consisted of a mixture of mystical and rational therapy. The prescriptions, as recorded on papyri, showed an amazingly complex *materia medica.* The weighing balance was known in Egypt as early as 1380 B.C. and some of the druggists were female. The *materia medica* included pills, suppositories, emetics, enemas, poultices, ointments, honey, beer, yeast, oil dates, opium and various lead preparations, parts of organs of various animals and castor oil.

Surgical management included the use of heated metal instruments to stop bleeding. The knife was used in ancient Egyptian surgery. It was made of stone in the earliest times, of iron as early as 1600 B.C. and latter of bronze or iron. Knives were used to cut hair, open abscesses and to remove tumors. Circumcision was done in Egypt as early as the fifth millennium B.C. Wounds were bandaged with linen dressings and impregnated with myrrh and honey. The Edwin Smith Papyrus describes the diagnosis and treatment of forty-eight injured patients grouped as listed below:

A. *Head*

Case 1. A wound in the head penetrating to the bone (incomplete).
Case 2. A gaping wound in the head, penetrating to the bone.
Case 3. A gaping wound in the head, penetrating to the bone and perforating the skull.
Case 4. A gaping wound in the head, penetrating to the bone and splitting the skull.
Case 5. A gaping wound in the head with compound comminuted fracture of the skull.
Case 6. A gaping wound in the head with compound comminuted fracture of the skull and rupture of the meningeal membranes.
Case 7. A gaping wound in the head, penetrating to the bone and perforating the sutures.
Case 8. Compound comminuted fracture of the skull displaying no visible external injury.
Case 9. Wound in the forehead producing compound comminuted fracture of the skull.
Case 10. Gaping wound at the top of the eyebrow, penetrating to the bone.
Case 11. A broken nose.
Case 12. A break in the nasal bone.
Case 13. Compound comminuted fracture in the side of the nose.
Case 14. Flesh wound in one side of the nose, penetrating to the nostril.
Case 15. Perforation of the bone in the region of the maxilla and zygoma.
Case 16. Split of the bone in the region of the maxilla and zygoma.
Case 17. Compound comminuted fracture of the bone in the region of the maxilla and zygoma.
Case 18. Wound in the soft tissue of the temple, the bone being uninjured.
Case 19. Perforation in the temple.
Case 20. Wound in the temple, perforating the bone.
Case 21. A split of the temporal bone.
Case 22. Compound comminuted fracture of the temporal bone.
Case 23. Slit in the outer ear.
Case 24. Fracture of the mandible.
Case 25. Dislocation of the mandible.
Case 26. Wound in the upper lip.
Case 27. Gaping wound in the chin.

B. *Throat and Neck*

Case 28. Gaping wound in the throat, penetrating to the gullet.
Case 29. Gaping wound in a cervical vertebrae.
Case 30. Sprain in cervical vertebrae.
Case 31. Dislocation of a cervical vertebrae.
Case 32. Displacement of a cervical vertebrae.
Case 33. Crushed cervical vertebrae.

C. *Clavicle*

Case 34. Dislocation of the two clavicles.
Case 35. Fracture of the two clavicles.

D. *Humerus*

Case 36. Fracture of the Humerus.
Case 37. Fracture of the humerus with rupture of the overlying sac tissue.
Case 38. Split in the humerus.

E. *Sternum, Overlying Soft Tissue, and True Ribs*

Case 39. Tumors or ulcers in the breast perhaps resulting from injury.
Case 40. Wound in the breast.
Case 41. Infected or possibly necrotic wound in the breast.
Case 42. Sprain of the sterno-costal articulations.
Case 43. Dislocation of the sterno-costal articulations.
Case 44. Fractured ribs.
Case 45. Bulging tumors on the breast.
Case 46. Abscess with prominent head on the breast.

F. *Shoulders*

Case 47. Gaping wound in the shoulders.

G. *Spinal Column*

Case 48. Sprain in the spinal vertebrae (incomplete).

Preventive Medicine was an Egyptian contribution. A true social medicine existed even in a rudimentary form. Hygienic regulations included instructions for the burial of the dead, methods of cleaning dwellings, diets, sexual relations and the requirement that only those animals could be eaten that were fit for sacrifice. Priests were obliged to cut their hair and to bathe. Newborn infants were wrapped in new white linen clothes. Complicated embalming techniques were developed to preserve the dead body according to the religious belief of life after death. The cult of the dead derived from this belief. It is apparent that the field of hygiene and social medicine in this rudimentary form was largely due to the prevailing religious orientation.

Among all the peoples of antiquity, the Egyptians enjoyed the reputation of having excellent physicians. These men were extolled by Homer and other ancient writers as a caste with special attributes. They were given priestly titles but were not necessarily priests. There were several medical schools. These were administered independently of the temples and were annexed to them as early as 4000 B.C. at Sais.

In 525 B.C. Egypt passed under the domination of Persia. This created a deterioration of the arts and sciences, including medicine, until the time of Alexander the Great two hundred years later.

The more vital part of Egyptian medical thought was transmitted to the Greeks and to Hippocratic medicine. Egyptian culture left a greater impact on civilization than did that of Babylonia because of the better preservation of its monuments of that culture—medicine, architecture, political sciences and religion.

*Education is a lifelong process in which the student can only make a beginning during his college course.*—Sir William Osler

# V Chinese Medicine

The youngest of the archaic civilizations (Fig. 8) originated in North China where three independent Neolithic cultures have been found. Crude gray pottery with pointed foot, red and black pottery similar to that found near Odessa and Susa, and thin black pottery, tentatively attributed to a Pacific civilization, are characteristic of all three of these earliest cultures.

Chinese medicine is said to have originated with three legendary Chinese emperors; Fu-Hsi, Shen-Nung and Huang-Ti.

Fu-Hsi created the philosophy of the Yang and Yin in nature in about 2900 B.C. Yang was considered to be the masculine element, representing all positive qualities, the heaven, sun, light, force, hardness, heat, dryness, the eyes, the left side and the dominant quality. Medicines were prescribed to excite the Yang. Yin was considered to be the feminine element, representing all negative qualities, the earth, moon, darkness, weakness, moisture, cold, ears, passive elements and the right side of the body. In Fu-Hsi's philosophy, the number five was considered to have great importance. Man, and everything else in the world, consisted of five elements (wood, fire, earth, metal, water). These five elements in turn corresponded with five senses, five viscera, five tastes, et cetera. Chinese philosophy of this period conformed to the religion of Lao-Tse in which man represented a microcosm in the macrocosm of the universe.

Shen-Nung is credited with originating Chinese medicine in about 2700 B.C. His contributions included: (1) cultivation of plants and the use of agricultural tools; (2) compilation of a herbal which mentioned one hundred remedies, and (3) introduction of the technique of acupuncture.

Huang-Ti was the author of one of the most ancient as well as one of the greatest medical works called the *Nei Ching* [Book of Medicine]. This is thought to have originated in 2600 B.C. Some historians believe that its origin is more recent.

Anatomy, diagnosis and therapy remained essentially unchanged during the centuries since their origin, except in those areas which were infiltrated by western civilization through the missionaries initially in the nineteenth century.

Anatomical studies are based on the ideas of philosophy because Confucius taught that the body was sacred and should not be touched. According to Chinese anatomy, the body has five organs to store nourishment (heart, lungs, kidneys, liver and

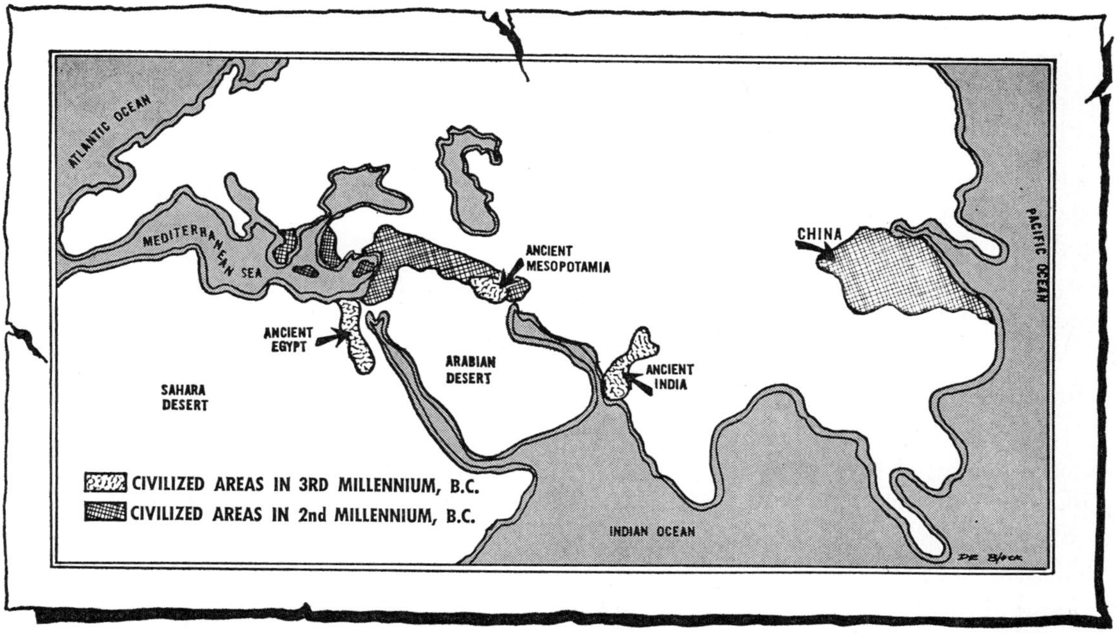


FIGURE 8. Archaic civilizations of the Second and Third Millenia B.C.

spleen) and five organs to eliminate and to be dependent (small intestine, colon, gallbladder, bladder and stomach). Each organ corresponds to an element, plant, color, season and has one or another of the organs as a relative. For example, the heart is considered to be the most important organ. Its mother is the liver, the stomach is the son and the kidney is its enemy. The "circulation" was not understood but was considered to be motivated by the Yang and to be completed fifty times every twenty-four hours. Dissection was first mentioned in the *Ling Shu* in about 1000 B.C.

Clinical diagnosis in Chinese medicine was related to the prevailing theory and methods of examination of the pulse. The human body and a chord instrument were considered to be similar and so harmony or discord in the body was felt to be discernible by the examination of the pulse. This examination would take several hours and the Chinese physician paid no attention to what we term medical history. The pulse would be examined in eleven places and three times each (light, moderate and strong pressure). Two hundred varieties of pulses were described and approximately twenty-six of these were felt to be indicative of impending death.

Medical therapy was regulated largely by the laws of Yang and Yin and included at least two thousand substances. Ephedrine, chaulmoogra oil, camphor, opium, sodium sulfate and many other medications were introduced. Organ therapy, including the drinking of blood was employed. Epidemics of smallpox were known and patients were innoculated against smallpox in the earliest times and yet this treatment is not believed to have been of Chinese origin. The crust of a pustule was pulverized and introduced into the left nostril for boys and into the right nostril for girls.

Surgical therapy in China probably began with the technique of acupuncture of Shen-Nung in 2700 B.C. This is perhaps one of the most interesting of Chinese surgical treatments and is still being practiced today in many countries, including the United States. Acupuncture consists of the introduction of a number of thin needles (cold or hot, silver, gold, steel or iron), from one to ten inches in length, into the skin. The purpose is to penetrate one or more of twelve imaginary channels which contain the two vital principles, Yang and Yin. These channels contain no blood but are believed to bear a close relationship to vital organs. Elaborate charts and details for the performance of acupuncture have been in existence since ancient times. Puncturing one or two of these channels is felt to remove obstruction and to allow the escape of bad secretions. The channels are believed to connect with three burning spaces located in specific places in the abdomen where the Yang and Yin are stored.

Castration was mentioned before 1000 B.C. and was used to provide eunuchs for the imperial court. Practical surgery for wounds was known in the third century B.C. Classic surgery for harelip was done skillfully and frequently as early as the ninth century. Deformation of the feet was accomplished by compressing the toes and raising the heel of each foot with bandages, beginning in the seventh year of life.

Hua-T'o was considered to be the greatest of the ancient Chinese surgeons.

*Nothing in life is more wonderful than faith, the one great moving force which we can neither weigh in the balance nor test in the crucible.*—
SIR WILLIAM OSLER

# VI Hebrew Medicine

THE HEBREW NAME for the land west of the Jordan River was Canaan. The term *Palestine* was believed to have been used for the first time by Herodotus, the Greek historian, and was derived from the word "philistine." This land was occupied in successive waves by people of Semitic speech, beginning with the Bronze Age in about 3000 B.C. The Semites, as these people were called, were greatly influenced by their neighbors to the east and south, Babylonia and Egypt, and still are.

About the fourteenth century B.C., the Joseph tribes settled the eastern delta of the Nile River at Goshen. They became enslaved by Pharaoh Ramses II. Moses, their leader, led a revolt from 1225 to 1200 B.C. and brought his people to the oasis of Kadesh. The kingdom of Israel was gradually and painfully consolidated by Gideon and his seventy sons, Saul, David, Solomon and many others, but finally passed under Babylonian rule in 605 B.C., to Persian rule from 538 to 332 B.C., to Alexander the Great from 332 to 323 B.C., then to the Ptolemies of Egypt and then to Rome.

Hebrew medicine was in the hands of a priestly caste and the history of medical thought in the ancient period of Israel was to be found among their religious laws.

Because of the efforts of Moses, Jehovah became the God of Israel, and replaced the Baals and took over their sanctuaries. He was proclaimed by Amos to be the international God of Justice in 750 B.C. This, as well as the elaborate temple worship, resulted in a new religion known as *Judaism.* This religion differed from those of other ancient peoples in that the Jews recognized one God and established monotheism as a basic concept of life.

Judaism considered God to be the source of health and of disease. He was believed to create diseases as deserved punishment for sins. This concept tended to subordinate magic practices and to concentrate all authority and power, including healing, in the hands of the priestly caste.

Ceremonies relative to purification, including baptism and bathing, were extended from the priest to all the people. This is partially the origin of the term "the chosen people." Caste was suppressed, the priests set themselves as examples for the people and became the custodians of the civil and penal laws. There were few professional physicians and Jewish physicians did not become prominent until the Middle Ages.

Social hygiene was a distinct contribution of Hebrew medicine. The religious laws included repose on the Sabbath as a divine decree and also the need for repose at determined intervals. Regulations were made for the bathing of lepers, for women in the menstrual period and pregnancy, for those having gonorrhea and circumcision. Prohibition of certain foods, ablutions before prayer, and restrictions relative to contagion were also established. The Hebrews obtained their ideas of contagion from Babylonia and blamed flies and rats rather than human beings as carriers.

Monotheism and social hygiene are the lasting tributes of the early Hebrew culture.

*Knowledge comes, but wisdom lingers.*—TENNYSON

# VII Medicine Of India

REMAINS OF A civilization dating back five to six thousand years have been found in India. Public hygiene in the form of a brick-built drain for the purpose of collecting refuse from homes and buildings along the street have been dated in the 3000 B.C. period.

Aryans of uncertain origin invaded India from the Iranian plateau around 2000 to 1200 B.C. and the history of India begins with these people. The Indo Aryans worshipped nature gods from 1200 to 800 B.C. These deities were similar to, but less personified than, those of Greece and Rome.

The caste system of India was gradually developed from 800 to 550 B.C. because of the desire of the priests and nobles to perpetuate supremacy and to diversify occupations. This system included priests, Brahmans, warriors and the commonalty. The latter group included farmers, artisans and slaves and the slaves were the first to be segregated because of their black color.

Buddhism was founded by Siddhartha (Gautama) Buddha (563–483 B.C.) as a part of a general reaction against Brahmanism. He taught that if an individual would pursue a way of life consisting of withdrawal for meditation and personal religious experience, and strict morality with self-sacrificial altruism, he could then obtain peaceful release and a state of Nirvana. Shortly after his death, five hundred disciples met in order to rehearse the doctrine and code of discipline. They established a monastic community and a means of propagation of the new religion.

Early Indian medicine was most systematic. Every pathologic concept had its place and every medical description was minutely described. Even in recent times the medical literature has held closely to these ancient models. Anatomical studies were not done because religious laws forbade contact with a dead body, so no progress was made in this direction. India of this period was not entirely isolated from the known world. This was a momentous period in history when Buddha in India, Confucius and Lao-Tzu in China, the prophets from Israel and the philosophers from Greece were creating the first great religions and philosophies of mankind.

Disease was considered to be due to abnormal relations among the three chief elements of the body (spirit, bile and phlegm) and to be caused by either physical or moral causes. The anger of the god Siva was believed to be the cause of "fever" which was notorious as the "king of diseases." Many of our common conditions have been known since these ancient times in India, including phthisis, smallpox and others.

The patient was examined with unusual completeness by the physician who utilized inspection, palpation, modified auscultation, tasting, notation of the appearance of the skin, tongue, form and extent of swellings, crepitus of fractured bones and the sweet taste of urine in certain diseases (diabetes?).

The *Ayur Veda,* literally "Knowledge of Life," is the name of the works that included the body of literature which gradually developed on the subject of medicine in India. Its most important medical contributions were the *Compendium of Charaka* and the *Collection of Susruta.*

Susruta was probably the outstanding medical personality in Hindu medicine. He was active between 400 B.C. and not later than 300 B.C., possibly shortly after Hippocrates. His work includes medicine, pathology, anatomy, midwifery, biology, ophthalmology, hygiene and psychology of medical practice (currently known as the art of medicine).

In Hindu society, as was the case in many of the contemporary ancient societies, punishment of wrongdoers was frequently accomplished by means of physical mutilation. Adultery was usually punished by cutting off the noses of the guilty parties. Such judicial mutilation may perhaps have been the chief cause for the introduction of plastic surgery.

The *Collection of Susruta* was mainly surgical. He elevated the art of handling a lancet or forceps to the status of a practical science and described some 125 surgical instruments. He described a rhinoplasty as follows:

Now I shall deal with the process of affixing an artificial nose. First the leaf of a creeper, long and broad enough to fully cover the whole of the severed or clipped part, should be gathered; and a patch of living flesh, equal in dimension to the preceding leaf, should be sliced off (from down upward) from the region of the cheek, and after scarifying it with a knife, swiftly adhere it with a bandage decent to look at and perfectly suited to the end for which it has been employed. The physician should make sure that the adhesion of the severed parts has been fully effected and then insert two small pipes into the nostrils to facilitate respiration, and to prevent adhesioned flesh from hanging down. After that, the adhesioned part should be dusted with powders; and the nose should be enveloped in Karpasa Cotton and several times sprinkled over with a refined oil of pure sesumum . . .

## SUMMARY

The medicine of ancient India contributed considerably in the field of materia medica and surgery and was fairly contemporary with Greek medicine. India played a role in Asia similar to that of Greece in the West. The medicine of India spread into Indo-China, Indonesia, Tibet, Central Asia, and as far as Japan, just as Greek medicine had done in Europe and the Arab countries. Hindu medicine tended to remain static because of its continuous connection with theology. The contributions of this culture were injected into Western medicine by means of the translation of the works of Charaka and Susruta into the Persian and Arabic languages about 800 A.D. during the golden period of the culture of the Eastern Caliphate. The accumulated knowledge of the Eastern Caliphate was not lost in spite of its destruction by the Mongols because of its transmission to the West by way of the Western Caliphate.

*Modern medicine is a product of the Greek intellect and had its origins when that wonderful people created positive and rational science.*
—Sir William Osler

# VIII Greek Medicine

The history of the medicine in early Hellenic culture cannot be separated from the history of its philosophy. Medical thought slowly sloughed off magical concepts and priestly dogmatism and became established with its base on observation. Tempered by criticism, also an eminently Hellenic trait, medicine became both an art and science.

The first great task accomplished by Greece was to unify its peoples. The first Greeks were an Aryan people from the plains beyond the Danube. The characteristics that later dominated all of Grecian civilization were developed by the civilization of the People of the Sea on the island of Crete between 4000 B.C. and 1400 B.C. It was here that the spirit of freedom of art, philosophic thought and medicine was developed, free, for the most part, from traditional rigidity, magic and priests. Cretan civilization spread to Greece itself in about 1600 B.C. and then rapidly declined on Crete during the next 200 years. This higher Cretan culture was adopted by the local princes and their people in Greece. Their way of life is well portrayed by Homer in the *Iliad* and the *Odyssey*. These poems were compiled over one thousand years before Christ and revealed the existence of an empiric medicine and one that was considered to be a noble art. The heroes of war were expert in medicine and surgery. Descriptions of traumatic lesions were realistic. In Homeric poems, one-hundred and forty wounds were described, with a mortality rate of 77.6 percent. The physician was held in great honor as "a man who was worth more than many others." Although anatomical knowledge was primitive, it was good on bones, joints and muscles. Life was considered to reside in the breath and the soul was thought to have its seat in the diaphragm.

Following the migrations of the Greeks and the establishment of city-states in Asia Minor, the Peloponnese, Athens, central and northern Greece, Sicily and Magna Grecia, medicine was also influenced somewhat by the Orient. The Greeks gradually changed by absorbing, with increasing frequency, their beliefs in incantations, superstitions, signs, demons and even new gods with attributes for healing. Soon particular powers were attributed to specific gods and particularly to Apollo and Aesculapius.

## THE CULT OF AESCULAPIUS

Apollo was considered to be the inventor of the healing art and Hygeia was the goddess of health. According to Greek legend, Aesculapius was the son of Apollo and of the nymph Coronis. Jealous of Coronis, Apollo had her slain with arrows. Their son, Aesculapius, was hidden from danger on a mountain by the centaur Chiron and was taught the healing art. Aesculapius became renowned for the performance of miracles of healing and became the god of medicine. This myth lead to a cult of divine medicine and to the worship of Aesculapius in temples throughout Greece. The cult of Aesculapius is believed to have originated in Thessaly where he was born and where serpents were frequent. Aesculapius is commonly depicted with a serpent entwined about his staff (Fig. 9). The cult spread widely throughout the Mediterranean basin and was introduced in Athens in about 429 B.C.

The temples of Aesculapius became medical centers where medicine was practiced exclusively by families who traced their ancestry to Aesculapius and who became a priestly group. This secret medical lore was later shared with others who took the oath that later became the oath of Hippocrates and the law for physicians. These temples were built in locations of natural beauty and suitable for the treatment of the sick. Hypnosis, diet, baths and physical therapy were the basic methods of treatment in these sanctuaries. The most splendid of the temples was located at Epidaurus where there were exercise grounds, a race track and a theater which would seat 20,000 persons.

All who came to invoke the intervention of Aesculapius underwent preliminary treatment outside the temple. This preparation consisted of purification by fasting, baths, fumigations and purgatives. Finally, they entered the temple and fasted, dieted and then were admitted to the ceremonies of the cult. These ceremonies consisted of prayers which suggested hope and which gave accounts of former cures. The patient was shown votive tablets which described medical cures of former patients. The patient was finally invited to the inner court of the temple and by this time was considerably relieved of pain and worry. Offerings were then made before the gold and ivory image of Aesculapius and the patient was induced by various methods to sleep at the feet of the statue of Aesculapius and to await the healing dream. The essential part of the entire practice was the dream or the hypnotic state. It was customary to dedicate to Aesculapius a representation of the part that had been cured (a votive offering) and money was thrown into the sacred spring if the patient could afford to do so.

During this period of psychotherapeutic temple medicine, the basis of scientific medicine was created by the early Greek philosophers. They sought to explain the universe by plain reason.

## THE EARLY GREEK PHILOSOPHERS AND MEDICINE

Both Plato and Aristotle have regarded Thales who founded the Ionian School of Miletus, as the initiator of philosophy. He lived from 639–544 B.C. and propounded the primary principle that water was the cause of all things. He and his followers attempted to explain basic facts whose comprehension was necessary for the creation of a biologic system. The Miletians and Anaximenes, equating the importance of winds in nature and respiration in human life, reduced the world to a single element; namely, air (pneuma).

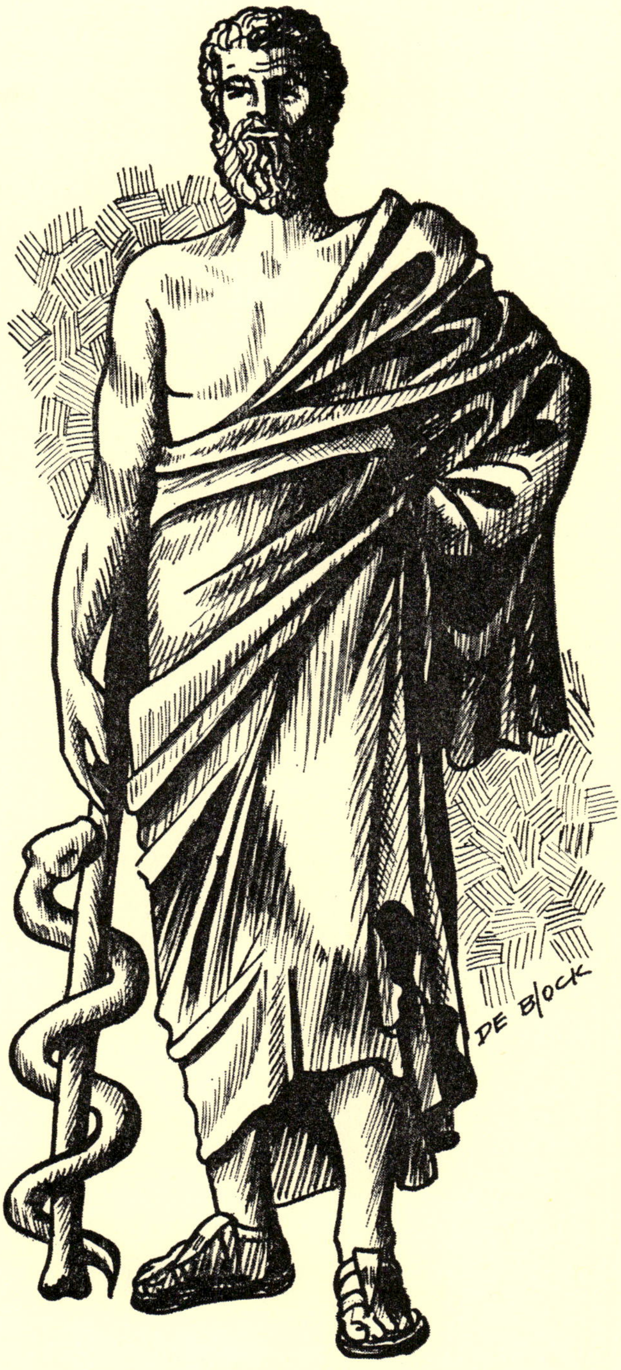


FIGURE 9. Aesculapius

Pythagoras of Samos (580–489 B.C.) provided a theory of harmony. He constructed an orderly universe based upon perfect numerical harmony and combined this concept with scientific experiments in acoustic and music theory. This became the basis of Hippocratic concepts of crisis, critical days and the healing power of nature. Pythagoras' pupil, Alcmaeon of Croton (about 500 B.C.), was the most distinguished physician of the pre-Hippocratic period. His medical school at Croton influenced the biological and medical concepts of the Pythagoreans. He was perhaps the first to practice dissection and he experimented on animals. He believed that the brain and not the diaphragm or heart was the seat of the senses and the center of intellect. He was the first to study the optic nerves and to distinguish veins from arteries. He provided a fairly important part of the origin of Hippocratic thought.

Finally, Empedocles of Agrigentum (504–443 B.C.) paved the way for the Hippocratic school with his four humors or elements (fire, water, air and earth). He considered the world and its people to be composed of these four elements and this concept dominated pathology for many centuries. He taught that the blood and heart were the seats of the vital spirits (termed *pneuma*) and he compiled some four hundred verses of dietary prescriptions into a volume.

The Greek philosophers, therefore, were responsible for initiating the humoral and the pneumatic doctrines which were to dominate medicine for many centuries to come.

More or less simultaneous with the temple medicine of the cult of Aesculapius and the developing concepts of the early Greek philosophers, an empiric type of medicine also developed. This medicine was practiced by military surgeons, court physicians and by wandering physician craftsmen. Flourishing schools of medicine developed. These were usually located in the great centers of commerce in the islands and coastal cities of Hellas and provided physicians for the purpose of practice in the armies, cities and courts. These physicians were independent of priestly medicine, which also continued to flourish quietly in the shadow of the sanctuaries. The empiric-rational school of medicine at Cnidos emphasized therapy based upon symptoms and diagnosis and used diet, herbs and drugs. A rival school was located on the adjoining island of Cos. Training at Cos included an art known as *pronoia* (the deduction of the past, present and future of an illness from the symptoms). Physicians were no longer dependent on a sanctuary and lived in closed intimacy with their masters and families like adopted sons.

## THE GOLDEN AGE OF GREEK MEDICINE

The golden age of Greece began in the fifth century B.C. (Fig. 10). Because of the decline of Ionia following numerous wars with the Persians, industry grew in Greece itself. Wages were low, shipping and agriculture were primitive and the economy was on a money basis. Pericles encouraged intellectual and cultural pursuits, extended Athenian imperialism and was involved in the Peloponnesian Wars. Herodotus and Thucydides wrote their immortal histories. Phidias' work with marble became the ideal of Hellenic beauty. Euripides and Sophocles stirred souls with their great dramas. The great Doric and Ionian buildings, such

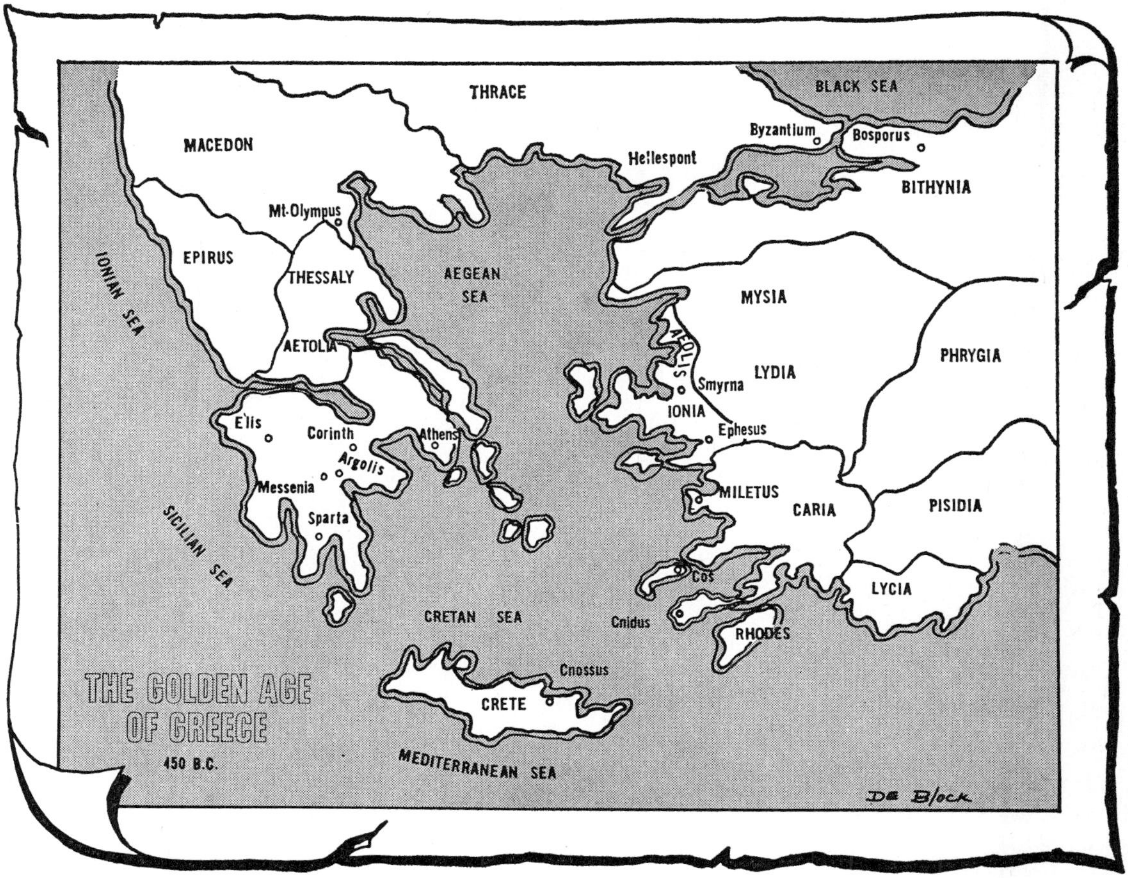


FIGURE 10.

as the Acropolis and Parthenon were constructed by Pericles.

The atomic theories of the philosophers Anaxagoras, Empedocles and Leucippus were believed to have solved the conflict against multiplicity. In the midst of all of this blossoming of Greek intellect, Hippocrates (Fig. 11) established himself as the most important and most complete medical personality of antiquity.

Hippocrates (460–377 B.C.. approximate) was born on the island of Cos. He belonged to the twentieth generation of Aesculapius and was a pupil of his physician-father. His studies took him beyond Cos to Asia Minor, Greece and Egypt. His main work was done, however, on the island of his birth. Four major elements were responsible for his great reputation.

1. *A principle.* Hippocrates taught that disease is a natural process and that symptoms are reactions of the body to disease. He further emphasized that the chief function of the physician is to aid the natural forces of the body. With this principle, sick people ceased to be considered as sinners and sinners began to be thought of as sick people. Hippocrates emphasized that the body possessed its own means of recovery and that a healthy man was one in a balanced mental and physical state because of complete harmony of all of the humors.

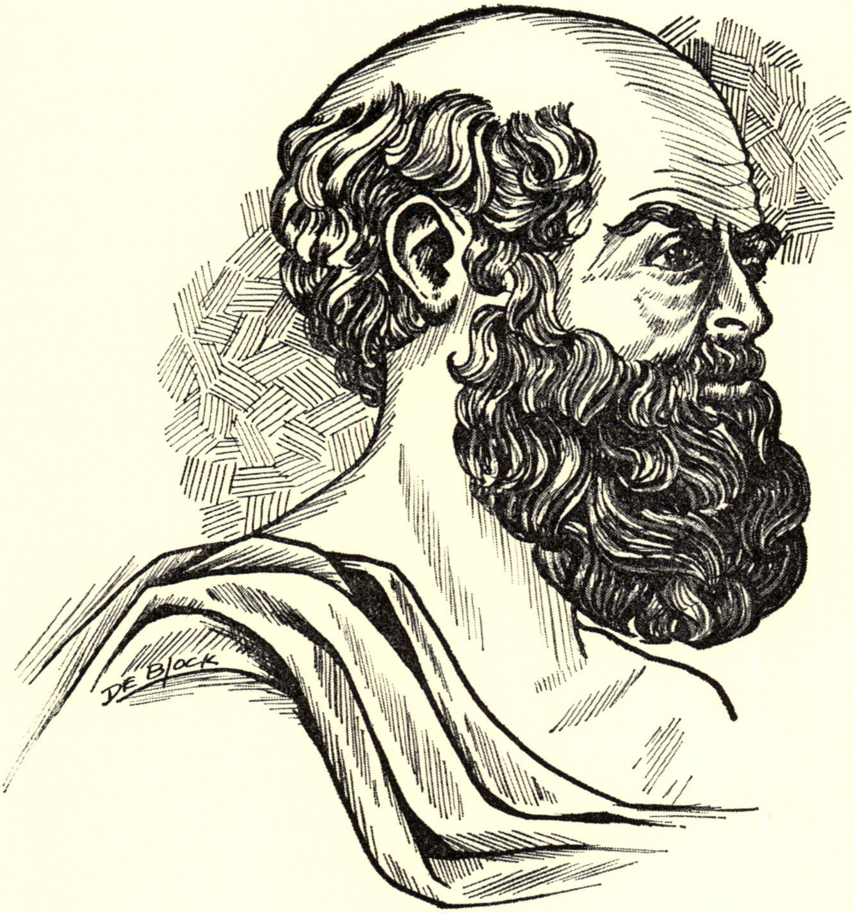


FIGURE 11. Hippocrates—"Father of Medicine."

2. *His writings.* The teachings of Hippocrates were compiled into written records. These writings may have been the library of the School of Cos. The *Corpus Hippocraticum* is truly one of the decisive writings in medical history and probably was written by Hippocrates, his colleagues, pupils and later disciples. It has been suggested that this work was actually accomplished during the third century B.C by Alexandrian scholars. Hippocrates and his disciples collected case histories in great detail. Some of the titles indicate the wide span covered by these writings, such as: On the Physician, On Honorable Conduct, Precepts, On Anatomy, On the Nature of the Bones, On the Humors, On Crises, On Critical Days, On the Use of Liquids, On Fractures, On the Seventh Month Fetus, On the Eighth Month Fetus, On Dentition, On Diet, The Prognostics, The Coan Praenotions, Of Praenotions, The Aphorisms, The Physician's Establishment, On Wounds and Ulcers, On Hemorrhoids, On Fistulas, On Injuries to the Head, On Fractures, On Reduction of Dislocation, On Airs, Waters and Places, and two of the seven books on epidemics.

Other books and writings probably came from others at the same time and at later periods and were included in the *Corpus Hippocraticum.*

*The Aphorisms* is the most famous of Hippocratic writings and is collected in seven books. For centuries, these writings were considered as the sum of all medical knowledge. Examples of some of these statements are listed below:

It is better not to apply any treatment in case of occult cancer; for, if treated, the patients die quickly; but if not treated, they hold out for a long time.

Diseases about the kidneys and bladder are cured with difficulty in old men.

In persons who cough up frothy blood, the discharge of it comes from the lungs.

Life is short, and the art long: the occasion fleeting; experience fallacious, and the judgment difficult.

3. *His pupils and disciples.* Physicians from all portions of Greece and the Mediterranean world obtained their training in the art and practice of medicine in one or more schools. The one established in the town of Cos was outstanding during the period of Hippocrates. The plane tree under whose shade he taught his pupils, according to legend, can still be seen. Hippocrates and the School of Cos created a number of outstanding individuals who then migrated to other centers to practice medicine and surgery with due recognition of Hippocrates as their authority and preceptor.

4. *His teaching of human compassion and ethical standards.* Hippocrates emphasized that a good physician must be one who was first and foremost a good and kind man. His teaching clearly enunciated the moral and ethical code of professional practice and created a new and reassuring image of a learned physician who was modest, humane and wise. The Oath of Hippocrates (Fig. 12) clearly indicates that the medical art is a doctrine of the initiated and that its chief aim is the cure of the patient without recourse to priestly rites or divine aid. He established that those who took the oath were physicians who practiced their art in freedom and taught in freedom—an ethical standard of highest order in an era prior to monotheistic teachings.

The theory and practice of Hippocrates and his pupils were fundamentally biological. They were based on philosophical concepts, particularly of Empedocles, and fortified by observation and experience. The body was considered to be composed of four elements (air, earth, water and fire). Each of these elements consisted of four qualities (cold, dry, hot and wet). There was no remarkable advance in anatomical knowledge during this period and Hippocratic teachings were based upon experience with animals. The physiology of the Hippocratic School combined the ideas of the Babylonian and Egyptian periods with those of the Greek philosophers and physicians. Heat was considered to be the essential factor of life. The pneuma was considered necessary for the maintenance of equilibrium of the body.

Hippocratic pathology was largely humoral and recognized four major elements as the basis of each organism and of life. These elements were: (1) blood, which comes from the heart and represents heat; (2) phlegm, which comes from the brain, generally diffuses and is cold; (3) yellow bile, secreted from the liver and representing dryness and (4) black bile, from the spleen and stomach, representing wetness.

# ΙΠΠΟΚΡΑΤΟΥΣ ΟΡΚΟΣ

I SWEAR BY APOLLO THE PHYSICIAN *and Aesculapius and health, and All-heal and all the gods & goddesses, that, according to my Ability and Judgment, I will keep this Oath and this Stipulation—to reckon him who taught me this Art equally dear to me as my Parents, to share my Substance with him, and to relieve his necessities if required; to look upon his offspring in the same footing as my own brothers, and to teach them this Art, if they shall wish to learn it, without fee or stipulation; & that by Precept, Lecture and every other Mode of Instruction, I will impart a Knowledge of the Art to my own sons, and those of my Teachers, and to Disciples bound by a Stipulation and Oath according to the Law of Medicine, but to none others.*

*I will follow that System of Regimen which, according to my ability and judgment, I consider for the Benefit of my Patients, and abstain from whatever is deleterious and mischievous. I will give no deadly medicine to any one if asked, nor suggest any such counsel; and in like manner, I will not give to a woman a pessary to produce abortion. With Purity and Holiness I will pass my Life and practice my Art.*

*I will not cut persons laboring under the stone, but I will leave this to be done by men who are practitioners of this work. Into whatever houses I enter, I will go into them for the Benefit of the sick, and will abstain from every voluntary act of mischief and corruption; and further, from the seduction of females or males, of freemen and slaves. Whatever, in connection with my professional practice, or not in connection with it, I see or hear in the Life of men, which ought not to be spoken abroad, I will not divulge as reckoning that all such should be kept secret. While I continue to keep this Oath unviolated, may it be granted to me to enjoy Life and the practice of the Art, respected by all men in all times! But should I trespass and violate this Oath, may the reverse be my lot.*

FIGURE 12. Oath of Hippocrates.

A defect or irregularity in this mixture was considered to be the cause of disease. Such defects could be brought about by various factors (congenital, accidental or determined by natural phenomena).

Hippocrates was the originator of climatology, which is the study of diseases which occur in a given locale in relation to its climate. He combatted the superstition that epilepsy was a "sacred" disease. He applied the term *phrenitis* to all diseases manifested by hallucinations or delirium. Malaria, pneumonia, pleurisy, phthisis, diarrhea, ileus, cirrhosis, mumps, diphtheria, erysipelas, gout, puerperal sepsis, cancer, epilepsy, paraplegia, tetanus, apoplexy and many other conditions were carefully studied and described.

The School of Hippocrates emphasized the importance of detailed observation of patients as the most fundamental obligation of physicians. Emphasis was made that the physician must know how to make an accurate prognosis of his condition in order to obtain the confidence of patients.

Hippocratic treatments were medical, psychological and surgical. The *materia medica* was large and was mostly of Cnidian or Egyptian origin and included purgatives, emetics, diuretics, narcotics and remedies for external use, including those for the eyes. The healing power of nature was stressed as was diet, gymnastics, exercise, massage and sea bathing. Purgative treatments of spring and fall were developed and were in great favor almost without interruption for twenty-five centuries.

Hippocrates and his followers knew of the advantages of pure or boiled water or wine in the treatment of wounds. There was still no understanding of asepsis. It was known that dry wounds were better than wet wounds. Bloodletting was rarely prescribed, except by those trained at the School of Cnidos. Obstetrics was done by midwives and pessaries were used in gynecology, sterility and cancer of the uterus. Surgical instruments included sounds, knives, trephines, the vaginal speculum, syringes, cannulas and forceps for extracting teeth. Operation for rectal disorders and for oral, nasal and eye conditions were done successfully. The treatment of fractures and dislocations was admirable for the period.

Plato referred to Hippocrates as the "Master of Medicine." Plato was twenty-four years of age when Athens fell to the Macedonians. Plato taught that man's immortal soul resided in the head while his mortal soul dwelled in his torso. He considered the heart to be the source of the blood, the liver to be the mirror of the soul and the spleen to serve for the cleansing of the liver. He conceived of the uterus as roaming in the body. Plato is believed to be the first to employ the term *anesthesia.* His pupil, Aristotle (384–322 B.C.), studied under Plato for twenty years, and he himself tutored Alexander the Great for a period of three years. Aristotle, too, followed the fundamental lines of Hippocratic philosophy. He became the physician to the Macedonian court. His studies were the beginnings of comparative anatomy and he made notable progress in embryology. He adopted the heart as the seat of emotions. He taught that the philosopher must begin with medicine and the physician must end with philosophy. With the founding of Alexandria at the mouth of the delta of the Nile River in Egypt (332 B.C.) by Alexander the Great, the center of Mediterranean trade, learning and medicine was relocated.

## MEDICINE IN ALEXANDRIA

After Alexandria was founded in 332 B.C., the Greek Ptolemy I Soter established the most famous library in the world. The Museum, or home of the muses, housed this library and it contained over half a million volumes. This center developed into the first great university in the world. It was complete with laboratories, a publishing house and even cafeterias. One of Alexandria's contributions to the history of medicine was the introduction of anatomic dissection as a means of study. The first foundations of pathologic anatomy and physiology were also created.

The Ptolemies administered Egypt as had the Pharaohs—as a state monopoly. They granted a privileged position to Macedonian settlers and to the City of Alexandria. Philosophers, physicians, artists and poets flourished. In this atmosphere, it was possible to obtain a fusion of Greek, Persian, Mesopotamian and Egyptian cultures. Mathematics was developed by Euclid and Archimedes.

As if feeling the need for filling in the gaps in the Hippocratic writings, the Alexandrian School devoted itself with enthusiasm to the study of anatomy, physiology and experimental pathology. Previously, the Greeks recoiled from touching a corpse because of fear of the spirit of the deceased and a natural terror of death.

Herophilos of Chalcedon was a leading figure in Alexandria and is considered as a founder of anatomy. According to Galen, he was the first to practice dissection on human bodies, although it is more probable that he was the first to do it in public. He studied the human viscera, described numerous organs and named the torcular Herophili (the confluence of sagittal and lateral dural sinuses of the head), the duodenum and the calamus scriptorius. His observations on the anatomy of the nervous system were notable. The work of Herophilus in anatomy led the way to the concept that diseases are not involved in any system of mysterious humors but have their origin in certain organs. Approximately a generation following Herophilos, Erasistratus (310–250 B.C.) not only dissected animals and human organs but experimented in metabolism. He is credited with discovering the tricuspid valve of the heart. The disciples of these two great Alexandrian physicians and scientists became founders of two sects, both lasting after the birth of Christ. Unfortunately, the pupils did not follow the outline or the example of their masters and carried medicine along a sterile pathway and became known as the *Dogmatists.* Contemporary to and perhaps as a reaction to its Dogmatists, the School of Empiricists developed in Alexandria between 270–220 B.C. This School maintained that only the practice of medicine can foster medical art and that theoretical discussions can be harmful. They regarded Hippocrates as their master. The doctrine of the Empiricists included three basic elements of experience: (1) personal observation; (2) tradition by the observation of others, and (3) analogy.

The political situation in Alexandria under the Ptolemies gradually deteriorated. With the suicide of Cleopatra in 30 B.C., the Hellenistic monarchy was ended and Roman domination began. Tragically, the great library and School of Alexandria were lost in the process. Fortunately, the accumulated knowledge had already been transferred elsewhere.

*With a half hour's reading in bed every night as a steady practice, the busiest man can get a fair education before the plasma sets in the periganglionic spaces of the grey cortex.*—SIR WILLIAM OSLER

# IX Etruscan and Roman Medicine

THE HISTORY of the people of Italy began in the Paleolithic Period. Bones from Liguria suggest that there were originally two races—Negroid or African, and Cro-Magnon or French. New races developed after the Ice Age, i.e., the Neolithic Mediterraneans appeared in approximately 2500 B.C., the bronze-using, Indo-European people in 2000 B.C., the iron-using, Terramare people in about 1000 B.C., and the Etruscans in about 900 B.C. The Greeks colonized southern Italy and Sicily in 760 B.C. and Rome was founded in approximately 753 B.C. We are concerned primarily with the Etruscan and Roman civilizations and their medical theory and practice.

## ETRUSCAN MEDICINE

The Etruscans probably came by sea from Asia Minor as a consequence of the breakup of the Hittite Empire, became a conquering minority and established themselves in Etruria just north of the River Tiber in about 900 B.C. They expanded until the end of the sixth century. A loose league of about twelve cities was established and government was by an aristocracy of princes. The Etruscan cities were fortified and Rome inherited most of its early culture from these people who were its first rulers. The chariot was introduced into Italy by the Etruscans who were a practical people and very much concerned with commerce. An Etruscan king started Rome's great sewer, the Cloaca Maxima, according to legend. Evidence indicates that the Etruscans excavated tunnels, leveled hills and drained swamps in order to combat malaria, which was common in this area.

Mythology also played an important role in the lives of the Etruscans as well as the Romans. The Roman theory of the *genius,* which is essentially that each individual is followed by a god who guides his star, is believed to have been derived from Etruscan mythology. Serpents were believed to be related to infernal gods.

The art of observing the viscera of animals, especially the liver, was of great importance to the Etruscans in their lives and in their medicine. The rite of Etruscan liver divination originated in Chaldea. Its transmitters were the Hittites who dominated the greater part of Syria and Mesopotamia during the second half of the second millennium B.C. This is the source of the bronze liver of Piacenza. This liver has been dated to the third century B.C. in Etruria and had the form of the liver of a sheep. It was divided into small compartments, each containing the name of the divinity either in abbreviation or fully spelled out. Each compartment of the bronze liver corresponded exactly to each of the regions of the heavens inhabited by corresponding divinity.

The thermal waters of ancient Etruria were known from very distant times for their benefits. Surgery and dentistry were practiced. Dentures containing gold work were of excellent quality. It was not until the second and third century of the Roman period that disease began to spread through the people in epidemic form. Etruscan culture became dead by the first century but it already made its contributions to the culture of the Romans.

The colonization of southern Italy and Sicily in 760 B.C. by the Greeks was also an important influence on the Romans. Although dominated by others, the Greeks managed to impregnate these areas with their culture. This lasted through the Roman period. The Greek heritage was disseminated widely as the Romans conquered the Mediterranean world and extended their empire.

## ROMAN MEDICINE

Most of the early Roman culture was inherited from the Etruscans who were its first rulers. Rome was founded about 753 B.C. as a union of small settlements on the seven hills overlooking the River Tiber and became the hub city of the future empire. According to legend, the founder was Romulus, the son of a princess and the god Mars. The Roman Forum was central to the hills of Rome and became a common meeting place where representatives of these early settlements also were able to develop a strong military alliance. From these small beginnings a mighty empire was to develop, to dominate the civilized world for over four centuries and to make particularly significant contributions in the fields of law and government.

The religion of early Rome consisted mainly in the worship of Mars. Originally, Mars was an agricultural divinity but later became god of war and of health. Ceremonials were simple and it was believed that by their proper performance the gods would be compelled to act. Failure to get results placed the blame on the ceremonial itself. The lives of the people and their medicine were dominated by these religious beliefs. Apollo and Mars, among many others, were the ancient protectors of health to the Romans. The Greek god of health, Aesculapius, assumed a similar role for the Roman people beginning in 293 B.C. At that time a severe epidemic was raging in Rome and all attempts to check it seemed futile. Roman legates were sent to the Temple of Aesculapius in Epidaurus. According to legend, a serpent made its way down the road and boarded the Roman vessel and entered the cabin of the legate and this was interpreted to mean that the god of health had entered the vessel and would give aid to the Romans. When the vessel arrived in the Tiber River the serpent is said to have swam to a nearby island and Rome was freed from the epidemic. A temple for Aesculapius was built later on this island.

Although it appears that there were physicians in Rome as early as the fourth century B.C., none were actually worthy of the name until the Greeks began to arrive in about 219 B.C. Roman medicine of this period was a mixture of magic and empiricism.

About the beginning of the first century B.C. the situation of the physicians in Rome was definitely established and this was largely because of Asclepiades. His preparation included the study of rhetoric, philosophy and medicine in some of the best schools of his time and particularly in Alexandria, which was the leading academic center in this era. A single incident is said to have brought him professional recognition in Rome. He interrupted a funeral procession, applied restoratives to the alleged corpse and was apparently successful in his attempt. He played a definite role in the evolution of the atomistic theory of life and in the intelligent interpretation of the doctrines of Hippocrates. Asclepiades maintained that the combination of particles moving on one another was brought about by means of small canals or pores in which the atoms were constantly moving. He taught that atoms in the atmospheric air were able to penetrate into the body by means of respiration and that the air and the blood were driven through the organism. Disease was believed to result if there was any disturbance in the movement of the atoms within these small pores. He is credited with originating distinctions between acute and chronic disease and with being the first physician to calm the insane with gentleness, music and sunshine. Asclepiades' maxim for medical care was *"Cito, Tute, Jucunde"* (Promptly, Safely, Pleasantly). His famous patients included Cicero, Crassus, and Mark Antony.

By the first century, the Empire was at its height and included Gaul, France, Spain, Greece, Asia Minor and Egypt. Unfortunately, Italy developed economic problems as the prosperity of her provinces increased and followed somewhat the pattern of her Greek predecessor. Although Stoicism was the dominant religion and philosophy of the Roman Empire, Christianity was spreading due to the journeys of Paul and others and in spite of the persecutions of the Christians.

The School of the Methodists followed that of Asclepiades and was the most important school in Rome at the time of the greatest splendor of the empire. The Methodists considered diseases to be due either to a state of abnormal tension or to a state of abnormal relaxation of the pores of the body with associated disturbance of the normal passage of atoms. Therapy was designed to restore the pores to normal. Surgical diseases were included in this system later.

The most celebrated physician of the Methodist School was Soranus of Ephesus because of his remarkable contribution to obstetrics and gynecology. Soranus began his work in Alexandria and then lived in Rome during the time of Trajan and Hadrian in about 100. He is credited with surpassing the medical knowledge of the Alexandrian School in his field. It was he who described the signs for telling the maturity of the fetus, to be the first to bathe the eyes of the newborn, to empty the bladder with a catheter before delivery of the child, to develop measures for the protection of the perineum during labor and to give rules for weaning and for contraception. Soranus is regarded as the "Founder of Obstetrics and Gynecology."

During the first half of the first century, two other schools were active in Rome in addition to a group of encyclopaedists who proposed to gather together everything that was known in their time about a given subject. The School of the Pneumatists followed a concept taken from the humoral theory of Hippocrates, i.e., the pneuma is the basis for health and is recognizable by the pulse. These physicians considered the study of the pulse, the use of proper diets, and the application of physical therapy to be the most important measures in medicine. The School of the Eclectics considered it to be their mission to free medicine from existing sects and to select the best concepts of each. The Roman Encyclopaedists were apart from the conflicting concepts and practices of the various Schools of physicians. These men sought to select, record and interpret the best in medical knowledge up to their time. The encyclopaedists included many patricians who were placed by their class above the practice of medicine but yet were drawn to it by their abilities to do library research. Aulus Cornelius Celsus and Pliny the Elder provided Latin classics of medical writing of this type. Neither man was a physician but both possessed vast culture.

Celsus wrote his book *De re medica* between twenty-five and thirty-five during the reign of Tiberius. This was the first-known attempt to compile a history of medicine, including the Greek and Alexandrian periods. This was the first translation of Greek medical terms into Latin. Celsus has been called "Cicero of Medicine" because of his fine literary style. He divided therapy into dietetic, pharmaceutic, and surgical. It was he who first described the four cardinal signs of inflammation (*rubor et tumor cum calore et dolore,* i.e., redness and swelling with heat and pain). Anatomy, dissection and autopsies were recognized in the Rome of this period. Celsus observed that a cut artery spurted blood and corrected Hippocratic teachings that arteries contained only air. Surgery as described by Celsus showed an advance in comparison to that of Hippocrates. Contemporary physicians ignored his work in that they were Greeks and looked down on the work of a Roman. Celsus' nomenclature actually dominated medical science for two millennia and his was the first book on general medicine to be printed. It was published in Florence in 1478, after having been rediscovered by Pope Nicholas V (1397–1455). The printing of this work is considered by some to be a significant contribution to medicine during the period of the Renaissance. Pliny the Elder (23–79) was considered to be the greatest of the Latin naturalists. His work, *Natural History,* included everything he had read or heard about plants, animals, races of men, anatomy, physiology, pathology, pharmacology, diseases and magical and rational therapy. He cited his authorities and named scores of the physicians of antiquity.

Three additional individuals were outstanding during this period: Rufus, Aretaeus and Dioscorides. Rufus of Ephesus (98–117) contributed an anatomical treatise and works on the pulse as well as descriptions of bubonic plague and traumatic erysipelas. He was first to describe the erroneous belief that the human liver has five lobes (like the pig). This mistake was perpetuated until the time of Vesalius. Aretaeus of Cappadocia was truly a Hippocratic type of physician who made model descriptions of diseases. It was he who observed that paralysis occurs on the opposite side of the body in cerebral lesions and on the same side of the body in spinal lesions. Dioscorides assembled all of the pharmacological ideas of his time in a treatise that was regarded for centuries as the leading text on the subject. He mentioned many new remedies and particularly those of mineral origin (lead acetate, calcium hydrate, copper oxide and other copper salts.)

During the second century, Stoicism continued to be the dominant Roman philosophy. The chief Stoics were the statesman Seneca, the slave Epictetus, and the Emperor Marcus Aurelius (161–180). The emperor was considered as the human counterpart of the guiding reason of the universe and to be obliged to rule for the good of his subjects. Law was dominated by the doctrine of the universal brotherhood of man, transcending the limits of city or station and emphasizing a humanizing trend. A municipal and provincial aristocracy appeared in the Senate and replaced the old Roman nobility because imperial service with complete loyalty to the emperor made this possible. The Empire approximated unification economically. Religious beliefs which were contrary to Stoicism were in disfavor and Christianity was considered to be only an oriental influence like the religions of the Egyptian Isis and the Persian Mithras. Medicine soon became dominated by Galen (Fig. 13) and was to remain so for fourteen centuries.

## GALEN (130–200)

Galen was born in Pergamum in Asia Minor (Fig. 14). He studied in Smyrna and in Alexandria. He was an outstanding student of the concepts and practices of Hippocrates. He prepared for ten years and then returned to Pergamum where he developed a successful practice. He came to Rome about 164, when he was thirty-four years of age and rapidly won attention for astute diagnoses. He scorned to ally himself with any of the quarreling sects of medicine and eventually became physician to the emperor.

The medical writings of Galen include eighty-three books that can be attributed to him, nineteen doubtful ones and fifteen commentaries on the Hippocratic text. These writings mark the culminating point in the ancient history of medicine. The most widely read of Galen's works was probably *De usu partium corporis humani* [On the Use of the Parts of the Human Body]. This rather amazing compendium of anatomy and physiology is considered to be one of the decisive writings in medical progress and indicates considerable justification for Galen's title as the "Father of Experimental Physiology."

Galen anatomy was better than any previous work even though Roman law prohibited the use of human cadavers for study. Galen obtained his information from apes, from the skeletons of criminals and from lower animals. He described the bones and sutures of the skull, traced some of the cranial and spinal nerves and made sections of the vertebrae and spinal cord. He described various muscle groups of Barbary apes in considerable detail.

Galen physiology followed his predecessors in the theory of *pneuma* as the essence of life. He knew nothing of the circulation of blood. It was his concept that the pneuma, the essence of life, consisted of animal spirits, vital spirits and natural spirits. The heart was considered to be the cen-

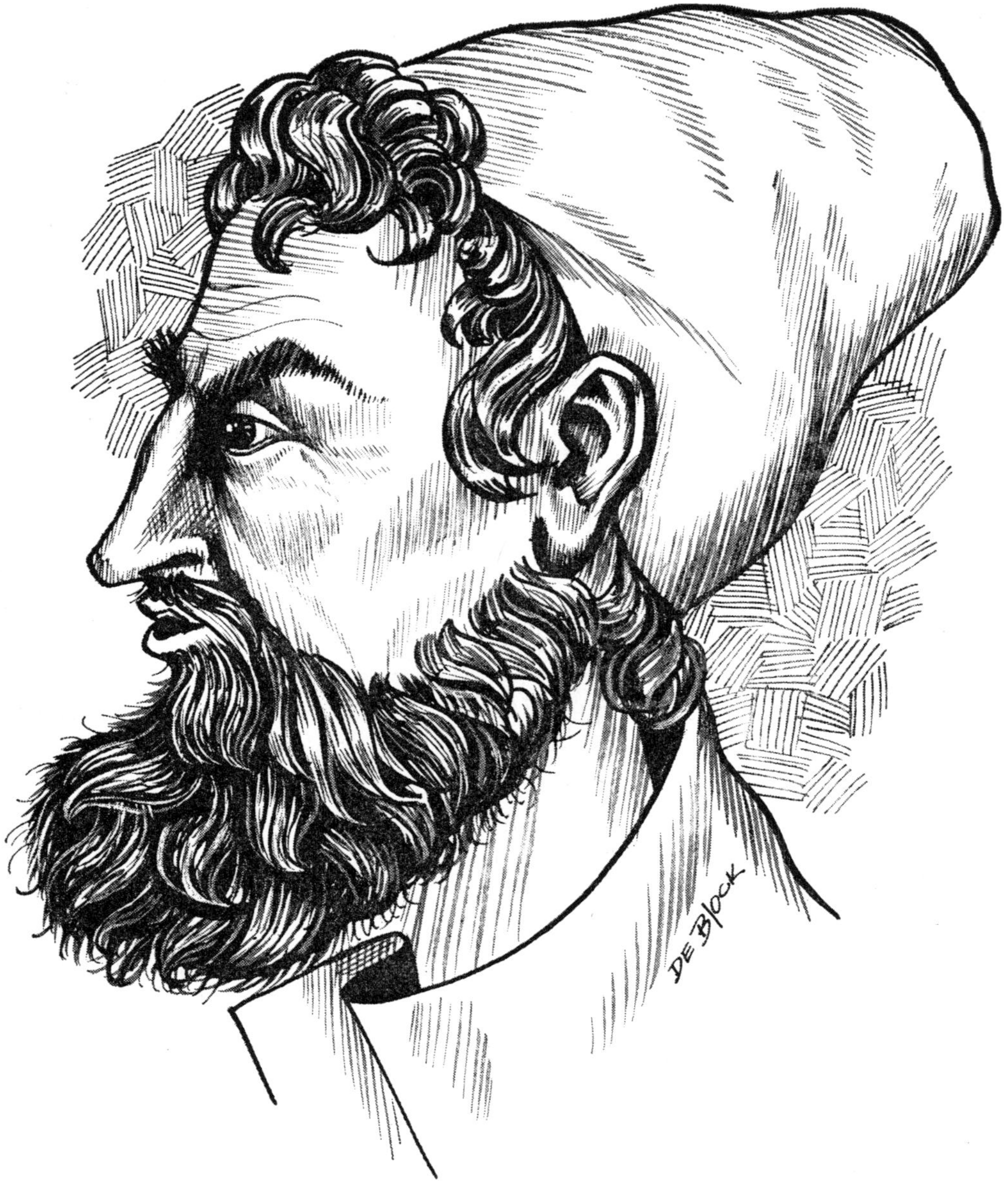


FIGURE 13. Galen—remarkable Roman physician.

ter for the movement of blood and heat regulation. The liver was considered to be the center for nutrition and metabolism and the brain for sensation and movement. He assumed that there was communication between the two ventricles of the heart by means of invisible pores and this mistake was perpetuated for nearly fifteen-hundred years. Thus, he had the animal spirits originating in the brain, the vital spirits mixing with the blood and the heart, and the natural spirits being developed from the blood via the liver. Galen believed that pneuma breathed by man returned to its source of

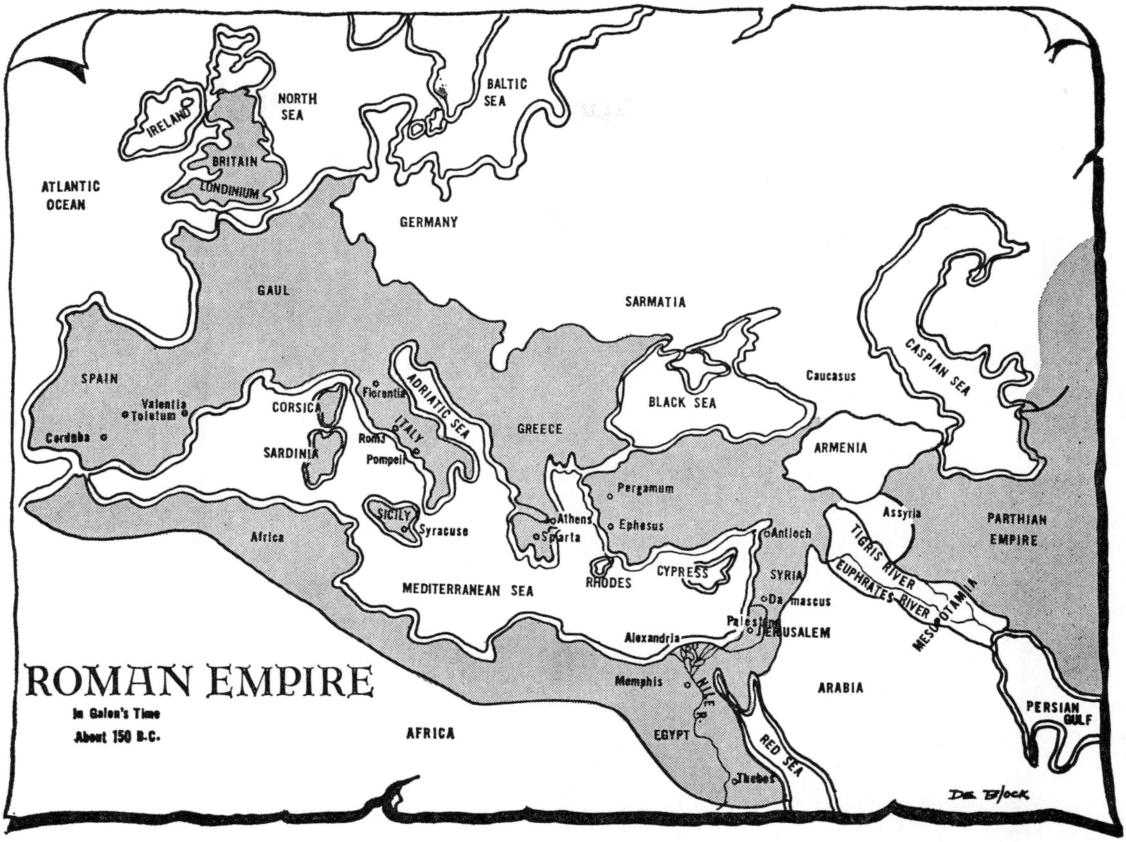


FIGURE 14.

origin at his death becoming a universal pneuma. He accepted that such a spirit turned into natural spirits in the liver, was distributed through the veins and transformed into vital spirits upon reaching the left heart and was then distributed through the arteries and finally became animal spirits in the brain and was then distributed through its "branches," the nerves. His concepts of physiology are depicted in Figure 15.

Galen was probably the first to produce cerebral lesions in animals, to establish a distinction between the lesions of the cerebral, cerebellar, brain stem and spinal levels, and to experimentally section the recurrent laryngeal nerve of a pig and of a dog to demonstrate the relationship of squealing and barking to this nerve. Two prevailing theories were disproved by the experimental section of the recurrent laryngeal nerve. Chrysippos of Cnidus had claimed that the voice came from the heart and Aristotle thought that the heart was the seat of intelligence and will.

Galen taught that the body is but an instrument of the soul. This concept corresponded with the essential features of Christianity and quickly received the support of the Church, and had much to do with explaining why all of the Galenical concepts were so rigidly held until the time of the Renaissance.

Galen pathology introduced an impor-

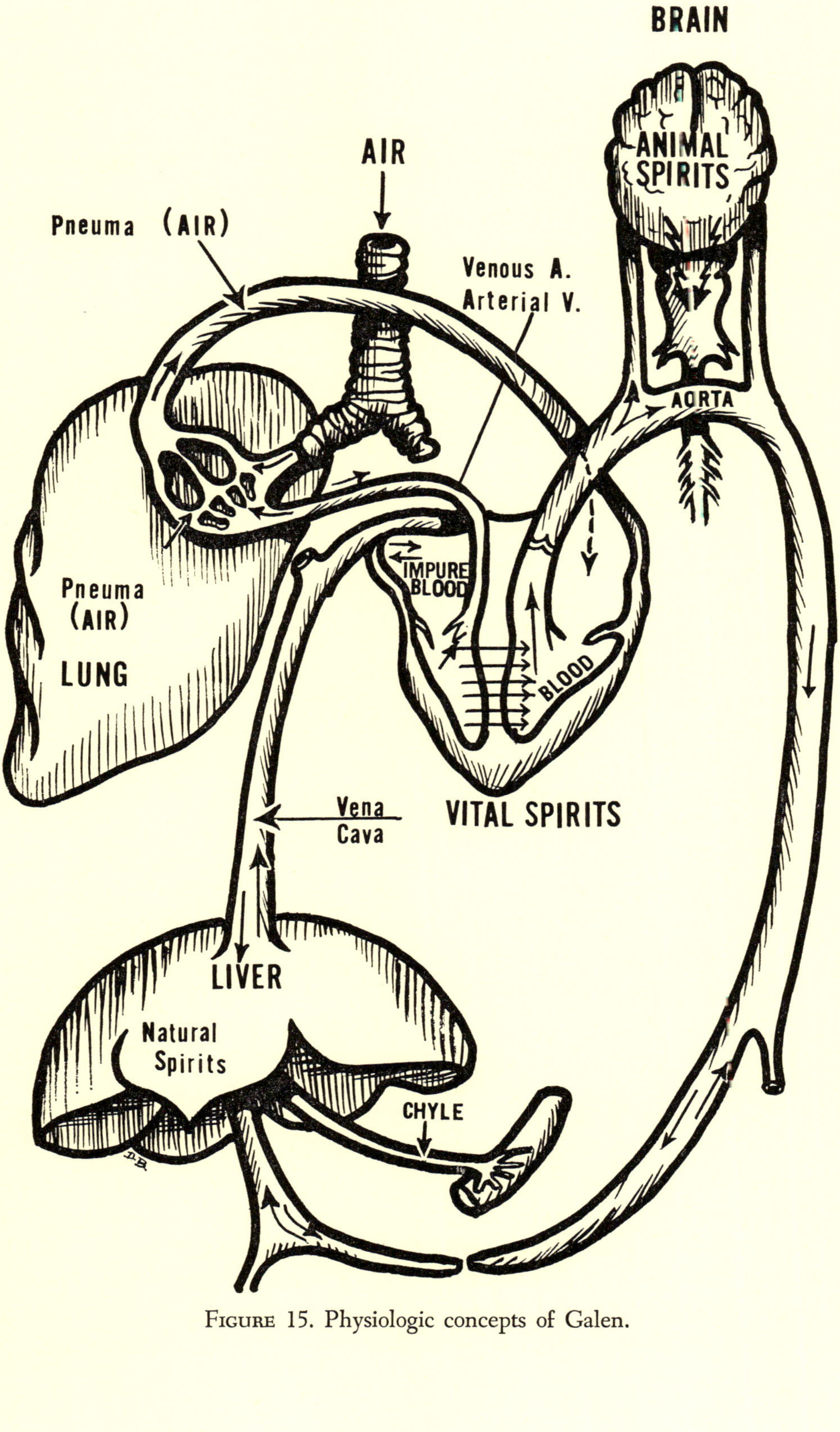


Figure 15. Physiologic concepts of Galen.

tant principle. Every alteration of function corresponds to a lesion in an organ and every lesion in an organ results in a change of function. He was the first to compose characteristic pictures of various diseases on the basis of this principle. He also supported the idea that suppuration (*laudable pus*) was essential to wound healing. This fallacy prevailed until recently.

Diagnosis by Galen was a fine art. He carefully examined his patients. He made excellent descriptions of sucking wounds of the chest, the infectiousness of consumption, and the problems of diagnosis with malingerers, hydrophobia, cholera and cancer. His diagnostic acumen was well shown in the case of a Persian sophist who had a sensory paralysis of the fourth and fifth fingers and one-half of the middle finger of the hand. Other treatments had failed and Galen asked about injury to the neck to find that the patient had fallen on a sharp stone receiving a blow between the shoulders following which he had immediately felt violent pain. Galen diagnosed inflammation of the spinal cord, ordered soothing applications and the patient recovered. His explanation was that because he knew that every nerve had a orgin distinct from others that the seventh cervical vertebral level was the area where this patient had been injured.

Galen's treatments were medical and surgical. The basic concept of his medical therapy was that of contrary measures. He applied heat for diseases that came from the cold and cold for diseases that came from the heat. He ordered evacuations in cases of plethoric conditions. He utilized diets, drugs, exercises, massage and climatotherapy. Bleeding held an important part in his therapeutics. The surgery of Galen made use of operations that had not been previously described including the resection of ribs in empyema and the resection of the sternum.

In total, Galen's work assembles the investigations of a gifted physician who utilized his great experience and practical observations in the practical sense. He also represents the speculations of a dogmatist. In his medical system, everything had its purpose and nature acts with perfect wisdom and does nothing uselessly. He made valuable discoveries but they were submitted to vain speculations in an attempt to coincide with Aristotelian philosophy. This, and his acceptance by the Church, made it virtual heresy to question Galen and thereby arrested progress until the anatomy of Vesalius in 1543, the discovery of the circulation of blood by William Harvey in 1628, and other notable events of the Renaissance era. The medical historian, Garrison, describes Galen as "the most voluminous of all the ancient writers and the greatest of the theorists and systematists."

Antyllos, who was active at about 150, surpassed Galen in the field of surgery and is considered as the greatest surgeon of antiquity. He was Greek and his works were lost except for fragments in the writings of Oreibasius. His greatest achievement was his work on aneurysms. For centuries he was the outstanding authority on the surgical treatment of aneurysms until his work was modified by John Hunter in the eighteenth century. He gave very precise directions for many surgical procedures including cataracts, tracheotomy, excision of scars, operations of fistulae of the bronchi, fistulae of the intestine and numerous conditions of the breast and abdomen.

## STATUS OF THE PHYSICIAN IN ROME

During the Republic, the practice of medicine was thought by Romans to be work for a slave. Greek physicians were generally resented or ridiculed. When the rights of Roman citizenship were granted by Julius Caesar to physicians in 46 B.C. the dignity and prestige of the practice of medicine was established. Thereafter, physicians became exempt from taxes and military service and were given salaried posts in the army and assigned to the care of private families.

Training of physicians for the entire Roman Empire was provided by a great number of medical schools, among which the most celebrated outside of Italy were those of Antioch, Lyon, Marseille, Saragossa, Athens and Alexandria. Near the end of the Empire, in the early part of the third century, the Emperor Alexander Severis (208–235) was the first to decree privileges for medical instruction, including anatomy of animals, medical botany, clinical instruction and examination of wounds. Those who taught in Rome enjoyed all the rights of citizens even if they were born elsewhere.

The decline of the Roman Empire and its complete collapse occurred during the third century. Medical factors in the form of five great pestilences contributed to this collapse. Each of these epidemics was accompanied by inundation and earthquakes and was followed by famine and drought. They were in:

1. 79, following the eruption of Mt. Vesuvius.
2. 125, following the destruction of crops by grasshoppers, when plague killed thousands of people.
3. 164–180, an Empire-wide epidemic of typhus fever.
4. 251–266, pestilence of Cyprian, smallpox.
5. 312, when a smallpox epidemic paralyzed political, social and scientific life.

Intellectual life was thwarted in connection with the absorption of the civilian administration by the military, by continuation of the emperor-worship test for Christians and their persecution, by frontier pressures by Germanic tribes, by the Persians, by economic collapse due to the heavy burdens of military taxes, and by a fatigue of spirit. The majority of the population lost interest and either accepted the invasions of the barbarians passively or welcomed relief from oppression.

When Diocletian became Emperor of the Roman Empire in 284, he desired to emulate Augustus and to revive the happy days of the earlier Empire. For practical administrative purposes, he divided the Empire into two spheres, Eastern and Western. Rule became absolute in view of the selection of troops without the consent of the Senate, and the military absorbed all functions of government. The Senators from the class of dominant, wealthy landowners and the rest of the population were crushed with taxes. Freemen were obliged to flee the country to enter monasteries or to become serfs on large estates. Diocletian took up his official residence in Nicomedia in the East in 285 and placed a military commander in Milan in the West to defend the northern frontier of Italy from barbarians. Rome then declined in practical importance except that the Bishop of Rome gained increasing influence. Thus, the center of political and medical leadership moved to the shores of the Bosphorus.

Persecution of the Christians continued in the West until 306 and in the East until 313.

Constantinus I the Great became emperor in 306, became a Christian in 313 and then proclaimed equal rights for all religions with restoration of confiscated property to the Christians. After the bloody and brutal military campaigns he reunited the Roman Empire under his sole rule from 324 to 327. Constantine realized that he would meet such opposition to the establishment of Christianity as the State religion in Rome that he decided on Byzantium as his capitol. He spent four years in building Byzantium as the strategic center of the East and dedicated it as his capital (later known as Constantinople). He made Christianity the official religion of the Roman Empire. He added schools in Athens, founded a university at Constantinople and extended the privileges of physicians and teachers throughout the Empire within the limits sanctioned by the Church. The gap between Rome and Byzantium grew wider until, by 395, they were permanently divided.

In summary, Roman medicine preserved the knowledge of antiquity because of the encyclopaedists, contributed considerable new information with the work of Galen, Soranus, Antyllos and others and developed a complicated sanitary organization due to the importance of medicine to the Empire. The writings of this era provided the means of transferring all accumulated information to physicians and scholars of later periods.

*A conscientious pursuit of Plato's ideal perfection may teach you the three great lessons of life. You may learn to consume your own smoke . . . we are here not to get all we can out of life for ourselves, but to try to make the lives of others happier . . . the law of the higher life is only fulfilled by love, i.e. charity.*—FROM *Aequanimitas* BY SIR WILLIAM OSLER

# X Byzantine and Monastic Medicine

THE END OF THE Western Roman Empire was brought about by invasions of barbarians in 476. Byzantium remained the major fortress of civilization during the next five centuries of the so-called Dark Ages. Alexandria, Antioch, Athens and Constantinople (Byzantium) became the four great centers of learning.

Medical practice was officially controlled by the Church in Byzantium, the sick were welcomed into the Christian community and medicine became dogmatic. It was based largely on a Christian faith which promised healing and redemption and appealed to the sick, sinful, despairing and the disinherited of the world. The early Christians transformed the temples of Aesculapius into churches and set up Christ as the healer of mankind. Patients were healed by the intercession of saints and church healing became as popular as the earlier temples of Aesculapius. Medical manuscripts of antiquity were preserved in the monasteries.

In many respects, the early Christians followed the rites of the Aesculapians. Cosmas and Damian were among the earliest Christian physicians. They had been martyred by Emperor Diocletian in the fourth century and became popular medical saints. Saints were believed to have powers to cure specific diseases. Saint Cosmas and Saint Damian were worshipped in Rome, Gaul, Greece, Asia Minor and at Byzantium. The well-known painting by Angelico and Gallego depicts a patient whose whole leg had been consumed by cancer. While asleep in the Church of Saint Cosmas and Saint Damian in Rome, these saints are said to have successfully replaced the cancerous leg with the leg of an Ethiopian so that after the patient had awakened from his sleep he found that he had been healed. Thus, temple sleep was practiced before a high altar and the patient dreamed of Christ and his saints and the dreams were interpreted by a Christian priest, rather than by the Aesculapians as in the past.

There was small opportunity for the orthodox physician in a society that believed neither in drugs nor in the study of the sick patient. Sickness and death were considered to be on the basis of divine visitation. There were also professional poisoners, dealers in spells and enchantments and sorcerers.

In spite of the dominance of the concepts of monastic medicine, there were a few unusual Byzantine physicians, such as Oribasius, Aëtius, Alexander of Tralles, Paul of Aegina and Johannes, who made contributions to medicine.

Oribasius was the most famous of Byzantine physicians. He was born in Pergamon in 325 and served as palace physician to the Emperor Julian who enforced strict licensure requirements for the practice of medicine. At the suggestion of Julian, Oribasius wrote his *Encyclopedia of Medicine* and preserved the works of medical writers of antiquity, many of whom would otherwise have been forgotten. He wrote with reason and judgment and in the best Greek tradition in an age which was dominated by superstition, magic and miracles.

Aëtius (502–575) was born on the Tigris, educated in Alexandria and was the first Christian physician of note. He wrote a resumé of all medical knowledge until the sixth century in his *Tetrabiblios* and served as physician to the Emperor Justinian. His work was characterized by keen clinical observation, Christian mysticism, incantations and great faith in Galen.

Alexander of Tralles (525–604) was said to have been the greatest scholar of medicine from the time of Galen until the age of the Renaissance. He was a member of a famous family from Tralles, near to Ephesus. He wrote in Greek and these writings were translated into Latin, Syriac, Gallic and North African. His influence on the Middle Ages was due to the Arabs and to Salerno where his works were translated, studied and admired. He was a follower of Hippocrates and Galen and also believed in incantations and amulets if other methods failed.

Paul of Aegina (625–690) was the last of the great Byzantine physicians. He was born on the Island of Aegina, practiced medicine in Alexandria and remained there after the Arabic invasion. His influence was great on the development of Arabic medicine. Of his seven books, his sixth was on surgery, his particular interest. He excised tonsils, resected ribs for empyema, used an expanding rectal and vaginal speculum, mentioned the ligature and described nasal polyps.

Johannes was a court physician at Constantinople during the later part of the thirteenth century. His work *On the Urine* was the best treatise on uroscopy that has survived from antiquity and contained the earliest account of hemoglobinuria. He also wrote *Functions and Disturbances of the Soul Spirit.* He attributed mental symptoms to bodily illness unlike his contemporaries who blamed evil spirits for such abnormalities.

Western monasticism was started by the Latin Fathers of the Church about 340 as a wide ascetic reaction against current corruption in life. It expanded rapidly in the sixth century and reached a chaotic condition which ranged from the most severe asceticism to the most lax kind of worldliness.

Scandalized by these conditions, Benedict withdrew to Monte Cassino. He founded a colony in this area between Rome and Naples in 529 and formulated the famous Benedictine Rule. This Rule dominated Western Monasticism for centuries and was a remarkable and characteristic Roman compromise adapted for the average man. It stressed labor in the open air and was much needed to revive agriculture in Italy. The order spread rapidly and became the chief instrument of the reform of the Gallic Church and for the conversion and civilization of England and Germany.

In the earliest periods of the Middle Ages, ancient manuscripts were copied and studied in the monasteries, thus providing for the survival of classical learning and classical science. This monopoly on learning and education in the monasteries was presently broken by the development of cathedral schools where, under the supervision of the bishops, young men could be instructed and prepared for admission to Holy Orders. Then came the establishment of universities under the influence of the Church at Bologna, Paris and Oxford.

The influence of this scholastic thinking was particularly unfortunate for the development of medicine because the study of diseases and of patients was neglected. It was the ambition of the learned physicians to study the writings of great physicians and to study commentaries on their works and not to study disease itself. The works of Hippocrates and Galen were tied to the philosophy and theology of Aristotle who became the towering intellectual personage of the Middle Ages.

The translations of the writings of Aristotle into Latin in the thirteenth century, and the works of the Arabian commentators, were the main factors in producing the scholastic period. The greatest minds of the age attempted to fuse all of knowledge into one comprehensive Aristotelian structure. This led to the fitting of all knowledge into tight compartments with sterility of creative thinking and lack of intellectual initiative, particularly in experimental science.

Albutt, the historian, has stated: "When Christianity became the state religion, it became narrower and harsher than paganism had been, and was used to stifle medicine and all the sciences." The role of "Byzantium in European civilization was almost wholly one of conservation or embalmment." When Byzantine civilization crumbled in the fifteenth century, after one thousand years, European medicine was already well-established and Arabic medicine had already made its contributions.

The Arabs were responsible for a new nation, for keeping alive the learning of antiquity and for making important additions to it from the second half of the eighth to the end of the eleventh centuries. They lacked the fetters which were fastening themselves on Western Europe and assimilated the remnants of Greek culture still present in the countries which they conquered.

*Wherever the art of medicine is loved, there is also love for humanity.*—HIPPOCRATES

# XI Arabic Medicine

MOHAMMED (570–632) founded the commonwealth of Islam in 622. During the next century, his followers had conquered half of the then-known world. He created classic Arabic by writing the Koran for his disciples in much the same way as Martin Luther did in establishing High German by his translation of the Bible centuries later. Arabic soon became the language of literature of the arts and sciences and of learned men in their writings and communications in the East as Latin and Greek had been in the West.

Interestingly enough, the greatest names in Arabic medicine were not Arabs but were Persians, Syrians, Jews and Spaniards. This state of affairs was presumably encouraged by the attitude of Mohammed who chose Harith, an unbeliever, to be his personal physician.

From its birthplace in Arabia, Islam spread first eastward into Syria, into Iraq and Persia and then westward into Egypt across North Africa and into Spain. Its spread was finally checked at the Battle of Tours in southern France by Charles Martel in 732. The Eastern and Western Caliphates were developed. Each had its court, centers of learning and actually competed with one another for prestige.

## THE EASTERN CALIPHATE

Jundi-Shapur and Baghdad were the centers of learning in the Eastern Caliphate.

The University at Jundi-Shapur in Persia was founded in 340 and later became the greatest center of medical teaching in the Islamic world. It was founded by the teachers and followers of Nestorios who was the deposed and excommunicated Patriarch of Constantinople. His heresy was that he believed that Mary was the mother of Jesus but not the mother of God. The most famous early teachers in the medical school were Christians. Greek texts were translated into Syriac. In that Nestorian missionaries had penetrated Persia, India and China, medicine of the Orient was also introduced. Bedside teaching was stressed in the hospital at Jundi-Shapur. This hospital, with its medical school, provided the beginnings of Arabic medicine. The last-known official record of the hospital occurred in 1869.

Baghdad became the medical center and intellectual capitol of Islam under Harum Al-Rashid who is perhaps more popularly known for his association with the stories of Arabian Nights. Mamun the Great continued this tradition. In the year 931, a Board of Examination for Medical Practitioners was established by royal decree. There were sixty hospitals in Baghdad by 1160 and the larger ones had extensive medical libraries. A House of Knowledge was erected near the Baghdad Observatory and was provided with a rich library. The Arabic medical authors of repute and merit numbered over four hundred in both Caliphates.

Hunayn (809–873) was perhaps the most celebrated and productive of the translators attached to the college at Baghdad. He produced more than one hundred original works including his *Ten Treatises on the Eye* which was the earliest systematic textbook in the field of ophthalmology. It has been said that he was paid in gold for his manuscripts according to their weight.

Jabir (probably ninth century) is famous as the "Father of Arabian alchemy." * He utilized Chinese ideas of chemistry, healing and the occult which he learned from Moslem missionaries. Arab chemists were familiar with and have been credited with the actual discovery of many of the ordinary procedures in chemistry, such as distillation, sublimation, calcination and filtration. Alchemy, alcohol, alkali and aldehyde are all Arabic words. The Arab pharmacists introduced many new drugs. Some of these are senna, camphor, sandalwood, musk, myrrh, nutmeg, cloves, mercury, syrups, julep, alcohol, aldehydes, solvents for drugs and rose water. They were also familiar with the anesthetic effects of cannabis indicas and hyoscyamus, when taken with wine or when inhaled. Jabir has been considered as one of the greatest personalities in medieval science.

Rhazes (865–925) was born in Persia and after preparation in music, physics, alchemy and medicine he became director of a large hospital in Baghdad in 907 and a court physician as well. His scientific output was extraordinary, including 237 works, of which half were medical. He is known largely through Latin translations. His *Treatise on Smallpox and Measles* was the first monograph written on the subject. His monograph, *Diseases of Children,* has led many to consider him as the "Father of Pediatrics." He was largely responsible for the use of mercurial ointments in medical practice and classified chemicals as "vegetable," "animal" and "mineral." As a great clinician and scholar, his descriptions of disease rank with those of Hippocrates.

Haly Abbas (ninth century) prepared his *System of Medicine* which was to be the first Arabic medical work to be translated into Latin. This manuscript contains an interesting criticism of ancient works and represents the best of Arabic medicine for clarity of expression and originality of viewpoint.

Avicenna (980–1037) represented the epitome of Arabic culture and learning (Fig. 16). He was a physician, philosopher, scientist, statesman and poet and considered to be a genius of the caliber of Leonardo da Vinci and Goethe. His *Canon* codified all existing knowledge, contained over a million words and was a required textbook at the University of Vienna five hundred years later. He attempted to fol-

* Alchemy is of Egyptian and Greek origin. Its fundamental premise is that all metals are essentially the same and that it should be possible to transform one metal into another. Gold was considered to be the purest metal and silver the next. Alchemists for centuries have eagerly sought the substance known as the famous "philosopher's stone" capable of transforming baser metals into gold.

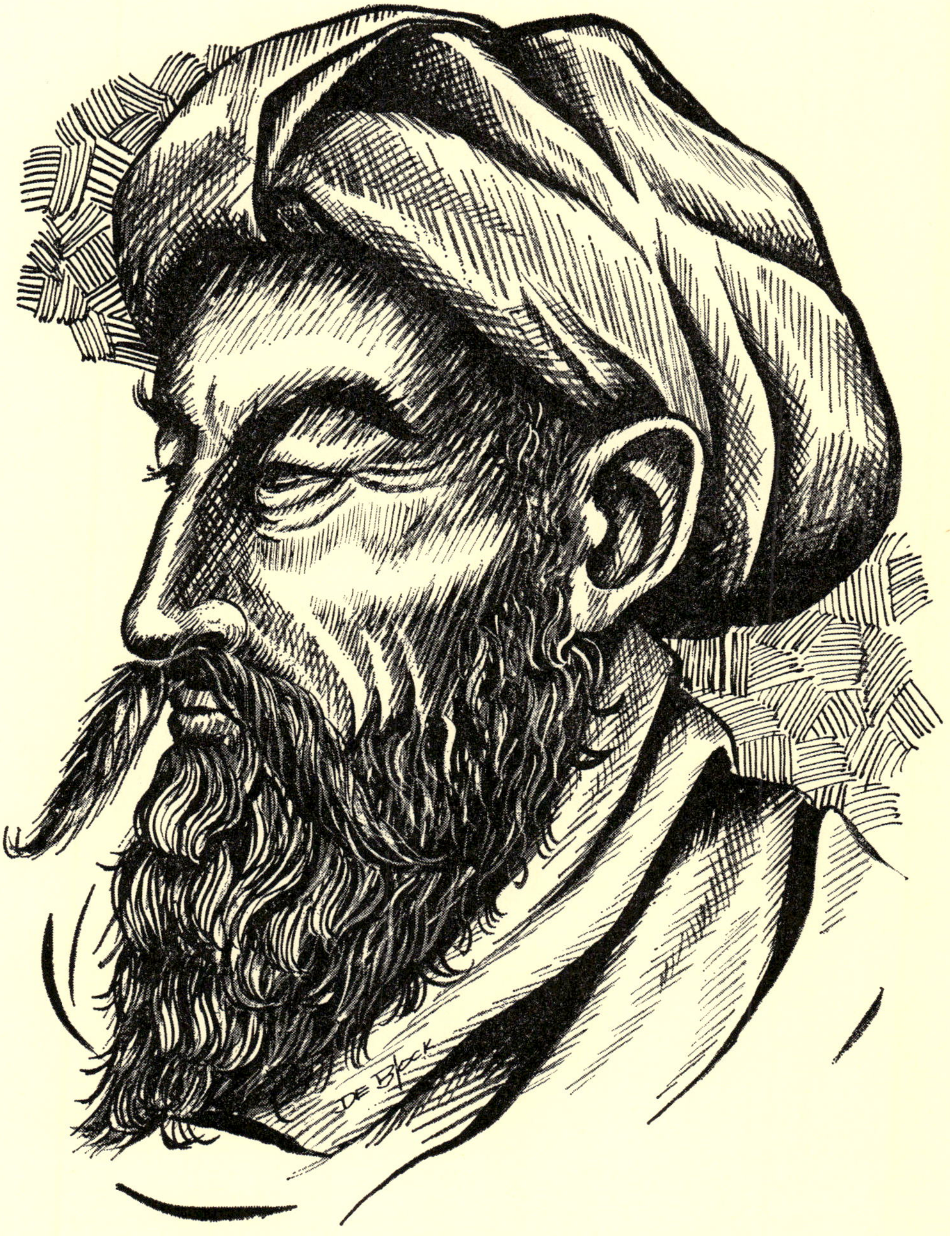


FIGURE 16. Avicenna—medical genius of the Eastern Caliphate.

low exact rules of logic and to fit each portion of anatomy, physiology, diagnosis and treatment into its proper category with mathematical accuracy. He added nothing new to the fields of anatomy and physiology because dissection was forbidden to Islamic physicians and he depended upon the Greeks for anatomy and Erasistratus and Galen for physiology. His diagnosis and treatment were complete and logical. The *Canon* was translated into Latin in the twelfth century, lasted for centuries and is considered one of the most influential medical writings of history.

Annafis (Ibn al Nafis) was an Arabian physician who lived in the thirteenth century. In his *Commentary on the Anatomy of Avicenna's Canon,* he pointed out that the interventricular septum of the heart had no pores and also gave the first clear statement of the pulmonary or lesser circulation. This work remained unknown to the western world for seven centuries, and others have generally been given credit for these remarkable discoveries.

## THE WESTERN CALIPHATE

Cordova (Chordoba), which is located in central Spain, became the most civilized city of Europe during the tenth century. It had a population of about one million people. The University of Cordova, which was founded in the eighth century, became a center of learning, even for Christians. The eminent medical men of the Western Caliphate at Cordova appeared long after Rhazes and Avicenna and had the advantage of possessing the accumulated knowledge of the earlier Arabian pioneers. The medical school at Cordova listened to Baghdad, but developed a preference for the concise, brief and exact, as contrasted to the expansive and hair-splitting of thought and diction of the East. It was also influenced by its immediate neighbors in western Europe. Four individuals were outstanding in medicine in the Western Caliphate, Albucasis, Avenzoar, Averroës and Maimonides.

Albucasis was born of Spanish parents in 936 and became the greatest surgeon of Islam. His major work was entitled *The Method* and was an encyclopedia of medicine and surgery in thirty sections. His last book, On Surgery, was the first independent work on surgery, the first illustrated surgical treatise and contained illustrations of more than two hundred surgical instruments. The first and longest section of *On Surgery* was on the use of cautery. He cauterized for headache, migraine, trigeminal neuralgia, apoplexy, hemiplegia, epilepsy, melancholy, cataracts, pediculosis, scrofula, hemorrhoids, sciatica, gout, hernias, leprosy, cancer and many other conditions. He described hydatid cysts and hemophilia. He also described a classic operation for cancer of the breast and warned against metastases. He advised ligation or cauterization of bleeding vessels and described fractures by reduction and immobilization. His work and the separate text on surgery fostered a tendency to divorce surgery from medicine. His followers were not judicious as he and cautery in surgery came to be employed excessively and improperly.

Avenzoar was the greatest clinician of the Western Caliphate. He was a vigorous opponent of the prevailing use of astrology and mysticism in medicine. His attacks on frauds and charlatans in medicine were beneficial. His aversion to Avicenna's *Canon* caused it to be followed less blindly but the by-product was an increased reverence for Galen.

Averroës attempted to build a system of medicine on the philosophy of Aristotle and some feel that this was written in the library rather than worked out at the bedside. His doctrine that the soul of man was absorbed into universal nature at the time of his death denied the doctrine of personal immortality which was accepted by both Moslems and Christians. He actually was close to the views of Saint Thomas in attempting to harmonize faith and reason but he and his followers were persecuted because of these doctrines. A School of Averroës appeared in Paris and in Padua. These philosophers attempted to reconcile Averroes with the Church dogma by the ingenious device of the "two truths" according to which a proposition could be philosophically true and theologically false or vice versa.

Maimonides (1135–1208) was Averroës' famous pupil. He eventually became physician to Saladin and published many works. His *Book of Counsel* was filled with sage observations and excellent advice and is the earliest-known example of this type of medical literature. He rejected rabbinical tradition and endeavored to reconcile faith and reason in his activities as a philosopher and religious teacher. He aroused much the same hostility in orthodox Jews that Averroes had created among orthodox Moslems. Maimonides is universally recognized in the Jewish world today as one of their great teachers.

Mongols virtually demolished the Eastern Caliphate. Baghdad was captured in 1258, when eight hundred thousand people were put to death and the literary and scientific treasures of centuries were almost completely destroyed. The Christians conquered the Western Caliphate. They did not destroy the culture of Islam but absorbed much of it and introduced it into Europe through Salerno and Montpellier.

## SUMMARY

For five centuries the Islamic Empire enjoyed the highest civilization and culture in the world during a time when Europe was floundering in barbarism and ignorance. Arabic medicine depended mainly upon the writings of Galen and not upon observation for its knowledge of anatomy. The Arabic physician took accurate histories of his patients and laid great stress upon the examination of the urine and pulse. His knowledge of drugs was extensive. He employed many drugs for the relief of pain, notably opium and administered mandragora for anesthesia for surgical procedures. Rhazes is considered as a peer among clinicians in all history. Avicenna is considered as one of the three or four universal geniuses of all time, with Leonardo da Vinci being his only rival. *Arabic medicine provided an effective link between the Greek and the Renaissance periods.*

*A university should be a place of light, liberty and of learning.*—BENJAMIN DISRAELI

# XII Medieval Medicine

THE CHRISTIANS had become strong enough by the eleventh century to begin a counteroffensive against Islam. The Great Crusades began in 1096. The eighth and last Crusade ended in defeat in 1270. The Papacy gained increased power and prestige by the unification of this group of quarreling and fighting princes into an army dedicated to the recovery of the Holy Sepulcher.

The crusaders were not suitable intermediaries for transmitting Islamic medicine back to Europe, but they did learn much from Islam about more refined living and hospitals.

## EARLY HOSPITALS

Hospitals were a major contribution from the period of monastic medicine but during that time were primarily refuges for the sick and poor with wards and apothecary shops and were not actually medical institutions. When Jerusalem was captured by the crusaders in 1099, they were surprised to find a Christian hospital open to receive their sick and wounded. This hospital was opened thirty years earlier by Brother Gerard in order to care for pilgrims to the Holy Land and was run by a small group of monks—the Poor Brethren of the Hospital of St. John. They were given buildings after the capture of Jerusalem and Brother Gerard formed his group into a religious order. They were called the "Knights of St. John" or the "Hospitallers" and were the first important Christian nursing order. They served the sick and wounded regardless of race or creed for eight hundred and fifty years, from the days of the Crusades to this century. Raymond Du Puy was their second master and taught the order the defense of the sick as well as nursing.

Saladin recaptured Jerusalem in 1187 and allowed the Knights of St. John to withdraw with their patients. They stopped at Tyre, Margot and Acre (with Richard Coeur de Lion). When Acre fell, they withdrew to Cyprus. In the meantime, the idea of hospitals was spreading to Europe. The Knights had seven hospitals in Italy as well as in Montpellier and in East Prussia. They moved to Rhodes from Cyprus. The Order of St. John now became a sovereign state with its own army, navy, diplomatic corps and laws. An immense hospital resembling a fortress was constructed on Rhodes but the Knights were obliged to leave Rhodes when it was captured by Suleiman the Magnificent. In that the island of Malta had been given to them by King Charles V, the Order of St.

John built a new hospital which became one of the most famous institutions of the world, the Order becoming known as the "Knights of Malta." The Hospitallers successfully defended themselves against the Saracens in 1565, lost to Napoleon Bonaparte in 1798 and then migrated to Rome where they still carry on in reduced numbers.

Arabic medical science eventually entered Europe through the wielders of the pen and the School of Salerno.

## THE SCHOOL OF SALERNO

The charming little city of Salerno was mentioned in Roman chronicles as early as 194 B.C. (Salernum) and is located approximately thirty-five miles southeast of Naples. Ancient Salerno can be traced back to the Greeks in the fifth century B.C. Because of its fortunate location, Salerno became a popular health resort and attracted both patients and physicians. The School at Salerno was mentioned as early as 848. According to legend, it was founded by a Jew, a Greek and a Saracen who lived in peace, harmony and brotherly love in spite of the prevalence of religious and territorial wars. The history of the School of Salerno has been divided by one of the most prominent authorities on the subject (Karl Sudhoff) into three periods:

1. From its origin in 848 to the arrival in Salerno of the Carthaginian monk, Constantine the African, in 1046,
2. The two centuries from the Norman conquest and the arrival of Constantine Africanus in 1046—the period of the greatest activity, and
3. From the first half of the thirteenth century on into a period of decadence.

Originally, lay physicians who practiced in the area had little learning and stressed experience. The School of Salerno gradually developed and fused the scholastic knowledge of the clerics and the practical experience of the lay physicians. The School maintained a close relationship with the Benedictine Abbey at Monte Cassino. A fusion of monastic and lay medicine provided stimulation for both institutions and by 1000, the School of Salerno had purely lay teachers (Fig. 17).

The Benedictine monastery at Monte Cassino was and is located on the same hilltop nearly halfway to Rome from Salerno. It served as a hospital and as a medical center preserving the remnants of classical culture and civilization following the destruction of the Roman Empire.

In a ninth century manuscript from the Benedictine Abbey at Monte Cassino, Sudhoff found directions for the *preparation of a soporific sponge:*

> Hypnotic Aid, that is a soporific suitable for those who are treated by surgery, so that asleep, they do not feel the pain of cutting. Rx: Opium ½ oz., Mandragora Juice 8 oz., fresh Hemlock Juice, Hyoscyamus 3 oz., together with sufficient water so that it forms a liquor, and then absorb in a fresh dry sponge and dry it carefully. And when thou wouldst employ this sponge, dip it in warm water, place it over the nose and cause the patient to breath deeply until he sleeps. And when thou wouldst wake him up, apply to his nose another sponge soaked with vinegar and thou willst end his sleep.

The School of Salerno was the first to employ *local anesthesia* for operations. Hyoscyamus and mandragora were made into a cataplasm and placed on the spot where an incision or operation was to be performed. This abolished sensation so that pain was not felt. (The formula for soporific mixtures is believed to have been of Arabic origin.)

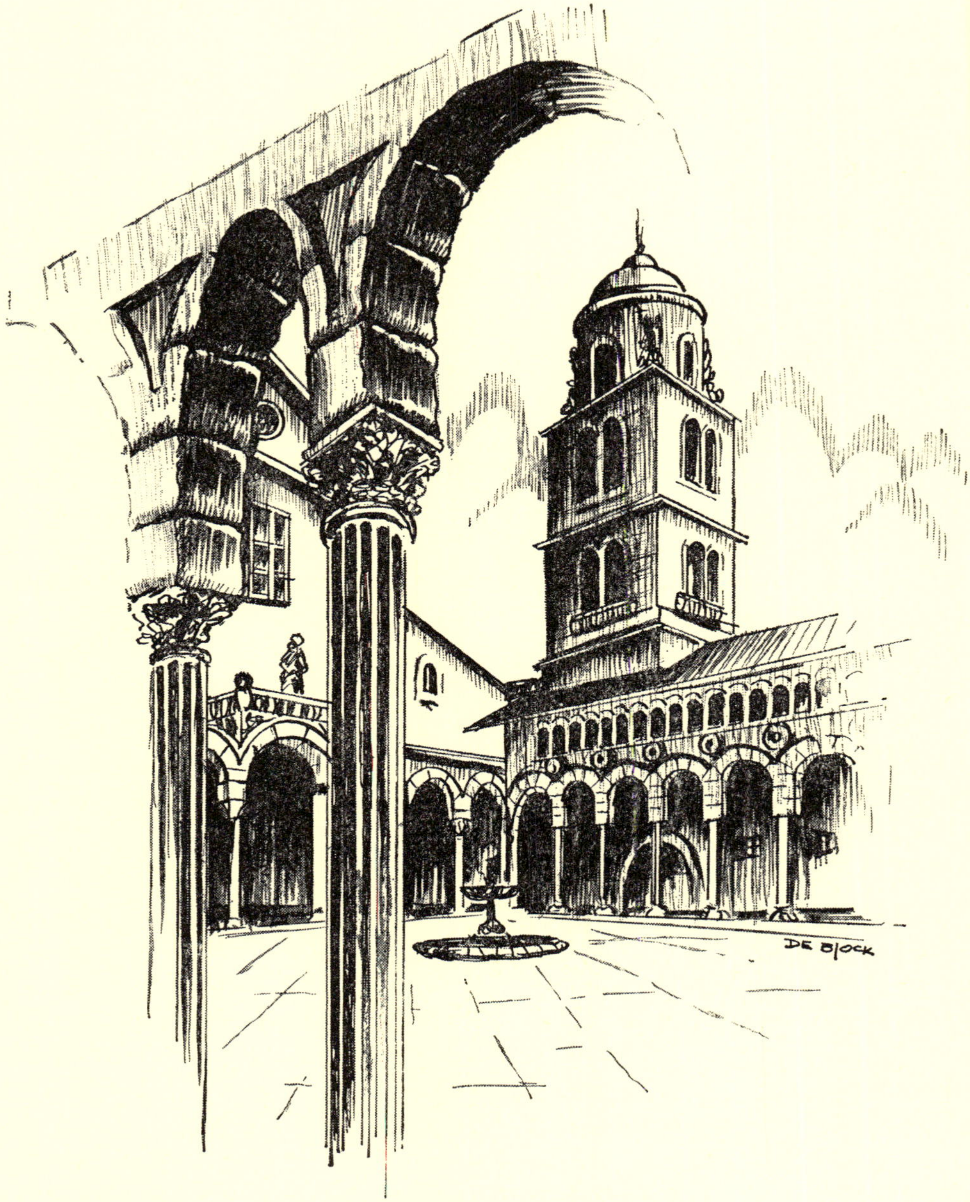


FIGURE 17. The School of Salerno.

The Normans conquered Sicily after it had been under Saracen rule for over two centuries and then captured Salerno from the Lombard kingdom in 1046. Constantinus Africanus (1020–1087) was secretary to the military commander of the Normans and was responsible for starting the flow of Islamic medicine into Europe. He was a native of Carthage and had spent many years in Baghdad and in other eastern cities learning the medicine and science of the Greeks, Babylonians, Indians and in perfecting his knowledge of Latin, Greek and Arabic. He was initially connected with the School of Salerno but eventually retired to the Benedictine Abbey at Monte Cassino to spend the remainder of his life in the translation of Arabic medical works into Latin. He is remembered as the "First Latinizer of Arabic Culture." *

The School of Salerno taught not only medicine but also philosophy, law and theology—the basic quartet of the university system. Several well-known books originated from members of this school. Gariopontus produced an authoritative text on therapeutics in 1050 (*Passionarius Galeni*). Nicolas Salernitanus wrote *Antidotarium,* a book on prescriptions. Trotula's book was the first in western Europe on the subject of obstetrics by a Christian author. This treatise, *Diseases of Women,* was a practical book describing the conduct of labor, the care of the newborn, the feeding of infants, the treatment of prolapse of the uterus and of uterine polyps. The text does not confine itself to obstetrics and gynecology but also treats epilepsy and diseases of the teeth and gums as well.

*Regimen Sanitatis Salerni* is probably the most interesting and famous publication associated with Salerno. The poem is made up of medical advice on health. This counsel was that currently given to patients in many parts of Italy and southern France at that time. One precursor of the time is the supposed letter on health written by Aristotle for his distinguished pupil, Alexander the Great. *Regimen Sanitatis Salerni* was written initially for the benefit of Robert, Duke of Normandy, son of William the Conqueror. Robert spent a year in Salerno enjoying himself while recovering from a wound in the arm and during this time his brother succeeded to the throne in England. In spite of this, most versions of the poem began with a dedication to the King of England. The *Regimen* was given later to many other patients as a health guide following their treatment at Salerno and was eventually translated into every language. The first English translation appeared in 1539 and was done by Thomas Paynel. The most popular English version was the work of Sir John Harrington who was the godson of Queen Elizabeth. Harrington's work appeared in 1607. He was also the inventor of a water closet which could be flushed.

Salerno's reputation as a center of medical learning apparently came more from the group than from any one individual with the possible exceptions of Roger of Palermo, Roland of Parma, Gilles de Corbeil and Gilbertus.

Roger of Palermo taught clinical surgery at Salerno for many years. *Roger's Surgery* was the first medieval textbook on surgery and dominated surgical teaching and practice in Europe for a full century. Although it was written in 1170, it was used at the new universities of Bologna and Montpellier. His text was clear, concise, practical and free from long verbose citations from the work of others. In considering fractures of the skull, Roger advised that a finger be inserted in the wound "because there is no better method of recognizing a fracture of the skull than digital palpation." He then describes removal of the fragment and placing a cloth between the dura mater and cranium with pressure to hold the scalp together and the use of a cloth dressing soaked in the white of egg. He also de-

* Gerard translated some seventy Arabic works. He had been sent to Toledo by Frederic Barbarossa in order to translate Avicenna's *Canon.* His translations were considered to be superior to those by Constantine.

scribed the treatment of nasal polyps, hemorrhoids, fractures of the jaw, intestinal anastomosis and bladder stones.

Roland of Parma reedited Roger's text in about 1250 and added observations of his own. He was Roger's pupil and later professor at Bologna.

Gilles de Corbeil studied at Salerno and went to Montpellier in 1180. His strong championship of Salerno and its Greek tradition made him unpopular because of the local Arabic influence and so he moved to Paris. He soon became the leading figure in medicine in Paris because of his writing and teaching and has been described as the founder of the Paris School of Medicine. He was appointed physician to Philip Augustus, King of France and later became a canon of the cathedral but never apparently was a priest. His medical works on the urine * and the pulse were standard reference for nearly three centuries.

Gilbertus (1180–1250) was educated in England but was taught medicine at Salerno by Roger and his associates and was possibly also a student of Gilles de Corbeil. He was physician to the Archbishop of Canterbury of England. He completed his *Compendium Medicinae* in 1240. This work included the medicine of the ancients and of his contemporaries but contained nothing original.

A regular curriculum of study was developed in the School of Salerno during the twelfth century. By 1224, Frederick II ordered that no one should practice medicine in the Two Sicilies without having passed an examination before the Faculty of Salerno. In a decree of 1240, it was stipulated that before starting medicine, the candidate should have studied logic for at least three years, and that he must study medicine for five years following which he must serve for one year as an assistant to an older physician. This decree established medical fees, required attendance to the poor and regulated the practice of pharmacy, including the purity and price of drugs and the relations between doctors and pharmacists. In its golden period, the school was held famous not only by medical people but also among the general public. Students came from all parts of the world. Once they had obtained their degree from Salerno, they were able to practice their profession in every country.

The School of Salerno began to decline during the twelfth and thirteenth centuries but during this period universities were developed in Italy, France and England and these institutions picked up the torch of learning, developed and subsequently have been emulated, for better or worse, elsewhere.

## EARLY MEDIEVAL UNIVERSITIES

The establishment of the universities was probably the most imperishable legacy left to us by the Middle Ages. The Latin word *universitas* did not have the modern meaning of a school in which all branches of knowledge were represented. It meant a corporation of masters or of students in the twelfth and thirteenth centuries. It becomes very difficult to fix definitely the period at which a university, in the modern sense, was founded because each formed slowly from groups of masters and students of theology, art, law and medicine.

The origins of several of these medieval

* During this period of nearly five-hundred years, pictures of physicians showed them almost invariably holding up a urinal to view because the urine loomed large in all diagnosis.

universities and the work of a few of their leading physicians contributed considerably to medieval medicine and future developments. Bologna, Montpellier, Paris, Oxford, Cambridge and Padua provided the beginnings for a series of remarkable accomplishments (Fig. 18).

## Bologna

Bologna is located between Florence and Venice in Italy. It started with a private law school and developed into a university in 1158, including a corporation of doctors who taught medicine. Some regard this university as the oldest in Europe. Its charter granted Bolognese students important privileges of freedom of travel and freedom from the jurisdiction of the civil courts. The students elected their masters as well as their rector. The professors were originally paid by the students for their instruction but were later paid by the city. The city was proud of its university and decreed a death penalty to anyone who attempted to move it elsewhere or to suggest to the students that they study elsewhere. The same penalty was decreed for any teacher who taught elsewhere without permission. Bologna was a university of students from the beginning.

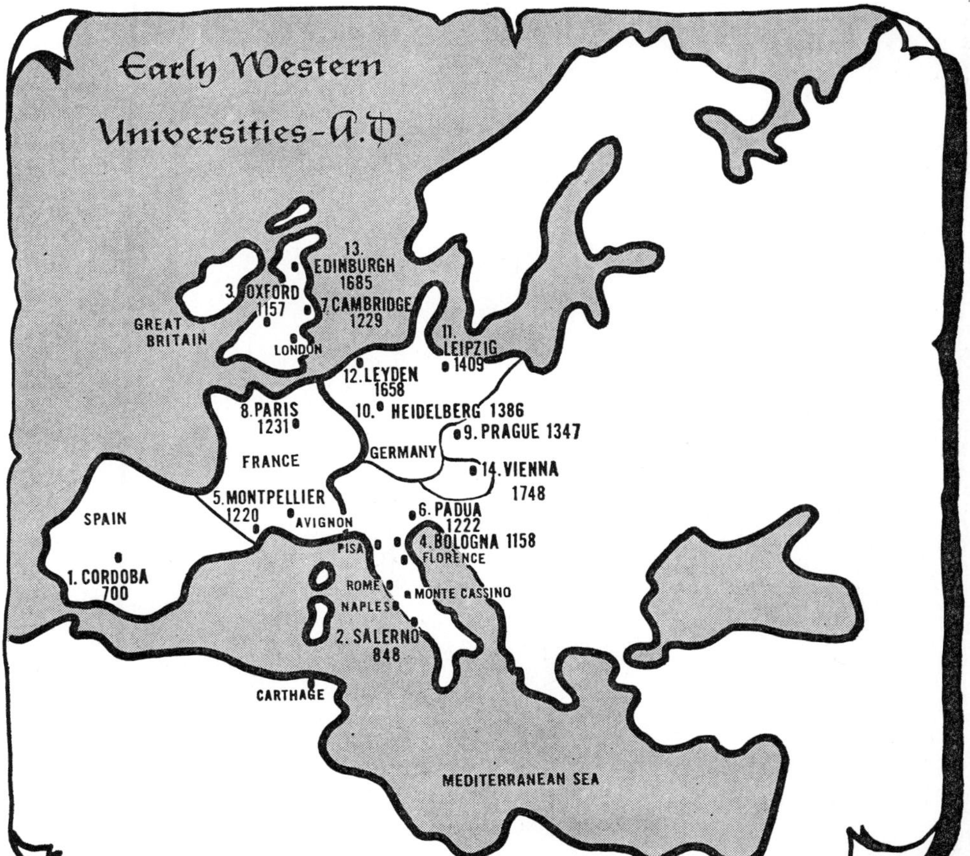


Figure 18.

Mention has been made that Roger's pupil, Roland of Parma, became a professor of Bologna after leaving Salerno and re-edited Roger's great text on surgery in 1250. Hugo of Lucca, who had been a surgeon with the Bolognese army during the Crusades was offered a very large salary to come to Bologna to be a public lecturer on surgery. He is known today largely because of his pupil, Theodoric.

Theodoric was a Dominican who became physician to Pope Innocent IV and later became the Bishop of Cervia. He lived most of his life in Bologna where he practiced and taught. Theodoric's *Chirurgia* was written in 1267. His writings record the surgical principles and practices of Hugo of Lucca.* He introduced a revolutionary treatment of wounds. He was concerned about the contamination of air of wounds and advised immediate closure with sutures in order to avoid suppuration. This concern and theory of preventing the formation of pus in wounds stands Theodoric as one of the most original surgeons of all time; Six-hundred years were to elapse before Lister elaborated on this theory and made surgery safer from infection. Theodoric credits the idea to Hugo. Writers on surgical history mention the "soporific sponge" of Theodoric as a landmark in anesthesia but Theodoric ascribes this also to Hugo. His famous pupil, Henri de Mondeville, spread these ideas to Paris.

William of Saliceto was said to have been the first to dissect a human body in Bologna and was considered by many to be the greatest surgeon of the thirteenth century. His famous pupil was Lanfranchi who became a leader of surgery in Paris along with Henri de Mondeville. The School of Surgery in Paris, therefore, stemmed directly from Bologna.

The School of Anatomy in Bologna became one of her greatest contributions and was linked to the name Mondino.

Mondino was a graduate in medicine from Bologna. After joining the faculty of the medical school in 1306, he devoted himself to anatomy. He wrote the first modern textbook on anatomy. His *Anatoma,* which was published in 1316, was a practical manual and had no illustrations. It rapidly gained a wide circulation, was written in rather poor Latin and was also full of Arabic terms. Mondino started his dissections in person and then turned the work over to his assistant so that he could mount his chair and explain the anatomy to his students. This method became the common practice for centuries and is depicted in the first anatomical text with illustrations, that of Johannes in 1481. The later editions show the well-known picture of Mondino presiding at a dissection. His knowledge was somewhat sketchy but he did sow the seed for further anatomical study. His pupil, Bertuccio, became the most famous teacher of anatomy at Bologna and taught Guy de Chauliac. De Chauliac carried the traditions of Bologna anatomy to Montpellier.

## Montpellier

Montpellier grew rapidly as a cultural and commercial center of importance in southern France near the Mediterranean Sea. Medical teaching was provided as early as 1000, but was apparently inferior to Salerno until 1181 when a decree was issued which granted anyone, regardless of nationality or origin the right to teach at

* Theodoric was possibly related to Hugo of Lucca, by spirit if not by blood.

Montpellier. The timing of the decree was right because of two important factors: (1) the beginning of the decline of the School of Salerno, and (2) the exodus of scholars from Cordova because of an edict that all must become Moslems. This brought Christians, Jews, Moslems and others to Montpellier and Arabic medicine was thereby reinjected into medieval Europe. The medical school was established by the Charter of Conrad in 1220. Cardinal Conrad had been delegated by Pope Honorius to supervise the teaching of medicine at Montpellier, to approve all of the professors and to see that no student of medicine could graduate without instruction from an approved master. The standards of the early teachers and students established the reputation of Montpellier and Arabic influence was strong for the next several centuries. Two of the outstanding personages of the Middle Ages were associated with this school. They were Arnold of Villanova and Guy de Chauliac.

Arnold of Villanova was born in 1235 and educated by the Dominicans in theology. He later studied the worldly sciences and became physician to popes and kings, Spanish ambassador to Paris and a student of alchemy. He assigned a leading place to the natural sciences in education and was an indefatigable experimenter. He maintained that "all true knowledge arises from the senses." He was in frequent verbal strife with his former teachers and was followed constantly by the vigilant eyes of the Inquisition.

Guy de Chauliac (1300–1368) carried the anatomic tradition of Mondino of Bologna to Montpellier. Dissections were permitted at Montpellier after 1340 A.D. He took Orders in the Church, became Canon in Lyon and also practiced surgery in that city. He later became physician to Pope Clement VI and remained there as physician to Clement's successors, Innocent VI and Urban V. He completed his *Chirurgia Magna* in 1363 A.D. This text was authoritative until the eighteenth century. He was a Galenist and did not follow Theodoric's ideas about wound healing. His teaching was based on surgical experience. His book contains extensive *materia medica* and also his description of the plague which visited Avignon in 1348. This picture of the Black Death is one of the best and most accurate in medical literature. He believed in astrology as did most of the learned men of his time. Although he did not teach in Montpellier, he made it famous as an alumnus. Fallopius called him the "Father of Surgery," as Hippocrates was the Father of Medicine. Many historians believed him to have been the greatest surgeon of the Middle Ages. The following lines tell something of his surgical philosophy:

> The conditions necessary for the Surgeon are four: First, he should be learned; Second, he should be expert; Third, he must be ingenious, Fourth, he should be able to adapt himself.
> It is required for the First that the Surgeon should know not only the principles of surgery, but also those of medicine in theory and practice; for the Second, that he should have seen others operate; for the Third, that he should be ingenious, of good judgment and memory to recognize conditions; and for the Fourth, that he be adaptable and able to accommodate himself to circumstances.
> Let the Surgeon be bold in all sure things, and fearful in dangerous things; let him avoid all faulty treatments and practices. He ought to be gracious to the sick, considerate to his associates, cautious in his prognostications. Let him be modest, dignified, gentle, pitiful, and merciful; not covetous, nor an extortionist of money; but rather

let his reward be according to his work, to the means of the patient, to the quality of the issue, and to his own dignity.

## Paris

Peter Abelard (1079–1142) was the eminent theologian and teacher who is given the chief credit for the founding of the University of Paris. The university was created by charter in 1231, from Pope Gregory IX, and included various schools, including medicine. By charter, the University of Paris was a university of masters where clerical control was complete, in contrast to Bologna where lay influence was predominant, including that of the students. Theology was the main subject and celibacy was enforced upon medical students and masters until it was abolished in 1452. The medical faculty remained under the control of the Church until 1595. The medical school did not achieve the wide reputation of Salerno, Bologna and Montpellier. Anatomy lagged behind, because it was not legalized in Paris until 1551 and the standards could not have been high because there were no failures on examinations of students for a century. Several outstanding men require mention, including Gilles de Corbeil, Albertus Magnus, Petrus Hispanus, Lanfranchi of Milan and Henri de Mondeville.

Gilles de Corbeil has been described as the founder of the Paris School of Medicine. He was born two years after the death of Peter Abelard and he brought the traditions of Salerno to Paris. He wrote and taught in Paris prior to the formal chartering of the university, including its School of Medicine in 1231. It is known that he was born in 1140, went to Montpellier from Salerno in 1180 and then to Paris. The exact date of his death is not known.

Albertus Magnus has been regarded as beginning the "Experimental School." He was one of the most learned men of the twelfth and thirteenth centuries. He was an influential teacher and prolific writer. He was an investigator with plants, animals, chemicals and minerals. He was canonized by Pope Gregory XV in 1622.

Petrus Hispanus studied theology, logic and medicine at the University of Paris. Originally from Spain, he advanced rapidly in the Church and became the first and only physician to be elevated to the rank of Pope. This occurred in 1276.

Lanfranchi of Milan was educated in Bologna and was a pupil of William of Saliceto. Like his teacher, he was a cleric and practiced both medicine and surgery with emphasis on surgery. He moved to Paris in 1295, taught surgery at the university and completed a textbook on surgery. Surgery was separated from medicine in France prior to Lanfranchi and was done primarily by itinerant unlettered surgeons. He deplored the separation of surgery from medicine and as an educated cultured individual was not without influence.

Henri de Mondeville (1260–1320) prepared in medicine at Paris and at Montpellier and then went to Bologna where he became a pupil of Theodoric. He remained Theodoric's faithful disciple. On his return to France, he became surgeon to the King in 1301 and remained in this capacity for the remainder of his professional career. He served Phillip the Fair and Louis X at home and at war. His wound treatment was strikingly successful. He attributed this to the methodology of Theodoric. He taught at Montpellier and wrote his *Chirurgia* which was the first French surgical text. This was circulated in many manuscripts but was not published until after the discovery of printing. If printing had been discovered earlier, and this book had been widely diffused, the whole course of French surgery might have been changed because of his remarkable section on wounds. Surgery in Paris lapsed after Henri de Mondeville. Disdain for operations grew and they were left to the laity. The chair of surgery remained vacant and in 1350, a statute required students to vow that they would not practice manual surgery.

*Addendum:* With the coming of Gilles de Corbeil to Paris and the injection of ideas from the School of Salerno, the faculty grew and lines became sharply drawn between physicians and surgeons. Surgical practice was actually forbidden to physicians and since the teachers of Paris, from 1231 until 1595, were under the control of the Church, they could not operate. The practice of surgery by monks was forbidden because of shedding of blood and surgery was relegated to persons of an inferior social status—surgical quacks and montebanks, for the most part. During these years, the Confrerie (College) of St. Come was founded by Jean Pitard (1228–1315). The college began as a mutual assistance society formed by those surgeons outside of the faculty of medicine. It was chartered in 1370 and slowly raised the status of surgeons. Surgery in Italy, by contrast, was highly regarded and the surgeons themselves were learned and cultured men. Unfortunately, the influence of Henri de Mondeville and Lanfranchi in Paris was mainly during their own time.

## Oxford

Oxford University was founded about 1167 by English students who migrated from the University of Paris because of an order by Henry II of England. He decreed all English students in Paris who were in Holy Orders to return to England or lose their support. This occurred during a quarrel with Thomas Becket who had the backing of the French king. Oxford was made a university of masters rather than of students and became a great center for classical learning during the Middle Ages. It never ranked as a medical center with the universities on the continent but did produce scholars whose investigations included medicine. Some of these individuals were Michael Scot, Bartholomaeus Anglicus, Roger Bacon and John of Gaddesden.

Michael Scot (1175–1223) was best known for his works on alchemy, astrology, physiognomy and on astrological medicine. Bartholomaeus Anglicus wrote *Concerning the Properties of Things* in 1250. This composition shows the first illustration of dissection in its French translation (1482) and in its English translation (1495). Roger Bacon was a Franciscan who wrote on gunpowder, the magnetic compass, the lens for reading, flying machines and is claimed by some to have predicted the discovery of America.

John of Gaddesden was probably the best-known English physician of the Middle Ages. He was born about 1280. His text, *Rosa Angelica,* was printed in 1492 and was the first to be printed by an English author. He was a cleric and had considerable scorn for lay practitioners and barbers.

## Padua

The university in Padua began in 1222 when a group of students from Bologna migrated to Padua as a result of the worst of many quarrels between the students and citizens of Bologna. Padua is located a few miles inland from Venice in Italy. The university was largely free from clerical domination and was much like Bologna and unlike either Paris or Oxford. It became a university of students. Padua soon rivaled Bologna and surpassed her except for historical prestige. The university enjoyed its greatest prosperity after Padua passed under the rule of Venice in 1405 and rapidly became the outstanding center of learning in Italy. Protestants and Jews obtained diplomas, indicating the tolerance which existed. However, in 1564, Pope Pius IV decreed that every scholar who graduated and received a degree from an Italian university must profess the Catholic faith and receive the degree in the Church. To avoid this regulation, Padua began to confer her degrees outside of the Church.

Anatomical dissections were practiced at Padua during the fourteenth and fifteenth centuries in an attempt to emulate the anatomical work of the Bolognese. Padua became the center of anatomical learning during the sixteenth century.

Distinguished teachers and pupils from the school of medicine at Padua were important factors not only in spreading the fame of the school, but in creating the Renaissance period in medicine and in laying the groundwork for modern medicine. Some of these remarkable men were Peter of Abano, Gentile, Linacre, John Caius, Vesalius, Fallopio, Marcurio, Fabrizi, Harvey, Santorio, Colombo, da Monte, Cardano, Fracastoro and Morgagni.

### Cambridge

Cambridge University was founded about 1229 by a migration of students from Oxford after a riot had occurred between the students and citizens of Oxford.

### Summary

The list of European universities during the fourteenth century is large. Most of these institutions were developed in Italy which was the undisputed center of culture and learning. Students from all of the countries of Europe were attracted there. They wandered from university to university because of the fame of celebrated teachers. Latin was the language of instruction and remained so for centuries. Language, therefore, was no barrier to learning even with the shifting of the centers of learning to universities outside of Italy. *The establishment of universities was probably the most imperishable legacy left to us by the Middle Ages.* This same period also witnessed two important but more temporary influences on medicine—astrology and epidemics.

## ASTROLOGY IN THE MIDDLE AGES

Astrology was regarded as a science on a par with law and medicine during the Middle Ages. The universities had chairs of astrology and it was as unusual for a doctor to doubt the validity of astrology as it was for a priest to doubt the authority of the Church.

The pseudoscience of astrology probably originated with the Chaldeans and spread through each succeeding civilization. It had reached medieval Europe mainly through the Arabians and came at a time in history that seemed psychologically right for such investigations. It was the common belief that man was the sole reason for the creation of the universe of which the earth was the center and that man's fate depended upon the heavenly bodies. Even the educated, therefore, concluded that a skilled astrologist could predict man's future. He had only to know the relationship of the planets to each other and to the signs of the zodiac. Astrology became important to governments, medicine and to all classes of people. The intriguing validity of astrology waned with the development of science during the next several hundred years.

## EPIDEMICS OF THE MIDDLE AGES

The epidemics of the Middle Ages had not only a profound influence on medicine but also on history (not unlike those epidemics of the Roman period). The diseases were different and in some instances were more devastating. These included leprosy, plague and the dancing mania.

### Leprosy

Leprosy was mentioned in the Brugsch Papyrus (2400 B.C.) and in the *Code of Hammurabi* (1900 B.C.). The disease was probably carried from Egypt by the Israelites. It was the subject of legislation by Moses. Confucius described the condition in China as early as the sixth century B.C. and it was also well-known to Susruta and to Charaka in India. Leprosy was mentioned by the Greek and Roman physicians during the first and second centuries of the Christian era.

The decrees of the Lombards, Franks and Charlemagne indicated that leprosy was becoming a menace to public health during the seventh and eighth centuries. It became pandemic during the eleventh, twelfth and thirteenth centuries. The leper was ordered to wear a black cloak, a tall hat and to carry a rattle. He was to sound his rattle if anyone approached him, in order to warn them. Such individuals were not confined, roamed the countryside in large numbers and were forbidden to touch anything exposed for sale except with a stick.

The decline of leprosy was partially due to severe protective measures and isolation, but primarily to the devastating effects of bubonic plague (the Black Death) which found its first victims among the weakened lepers. The disease was rarely seen after the fifteenth and sixteenth centuries.

### Plague

Bubonic plague (the Black Death) produced devastating effects on the people and their institutions during medieval centuries. Plague first appeared in China in 1334 and spread westward along the great trade routes. Twelve Genoese ships, which had come from Constantinople, apparently carried the disease to Sicily in October, 1347, then to Genoa and to all parts of Italy. Two thirds of the population of Florence died because of plague. The ships touched at Marseilles and the Black Death appeared in nearby Avignon in 1348. Pope Clement VI ordered the bodies of the victims to be examined after death and Guy de Chauliac, who was his physician, left excellent descriptions of the disease. The cause of plague was felt to be due to a combination of the conjunction of Saturn, Jupiter and Mars and the debility of those attacked. Some believed that the Jews had poisoned the people or had killed them and persecution of the Jews began in Europe in many places. All of the well-known Jews in several cities were seized, herded into a wooden building and burned. Two thousand Jews were hanged in Strassburg. Pope Clement VI declared the Jews to be innocent. The total number of victims of the plague itself was estimated to be 42,836,486 persons.

The physicians did not deny the astrological origin but were convinced that the disease was contagious. They isolated the victims from others and established the first quarantine of ships in Venice in 1377. The quarantine of ships became standard in most ports thereafter. Large fires were built in the vicinity where plague was known, in order to purify the air.

The impact of the Black Death was immense. The physicians of the period were helpless against it and the people sought supernatural aid. St. Sebastian and St. Roch became plague-saints. Half of the clergy of the Church were destroyed and their places were usually filled by men and youths with inferior training. The people saw their priests perish like themselves and they lost faith in the Church. Drinking, carousing and other excesses were uncontrolled. Plague probably played a dominating role in the abolition of serfdom and was one of the chief causes of economic upheaval in the Middle Ages. Thousands of landowners died, property changed hands rapidly and much litigation became necessary. Lawyers were almost unknown in countries such as England at this time but now appeared in large numbers. With the death of millions of workers, there was a shortage of labor and a rise in wages. The Black Death has been described by some to have contributed considerably as an important cause in the breakdown of the feudal system and in the establishment of the Reformation.

### Dancing Mania

As early as 1374, large crowds of men and women seemed to become obsessed by a strange mania. They first appeared on the streets of Aachen, formed circles, hand-in-hand, and danced wildly for hours. They seemed oblivious to the jeers and taunts of onlookers. This mania spread from town to town. Disorder resulted and it was necessary for the town council in Strassburg to take active measures to aid the afflicted by dividing them into small groups. They were sent to the chapels of St. Vitus where priests, by means of masses and other religious observances, apparently cured them of their strange affliction. The Dancing Mania appeared in Germany during the time of the misery that was produced by the Black Death and was called the Dance of St. John or of St. Vitus. It was labeled Chorea St. Vitii or St. Vitus dance by Paracelsus. This was a mass hysteria, rather than the disease we now know as St. Vitus dance or Sydenham's chorea.

## CONCLUSIONS

The Middle Ages was a time in history that was sufficiently constructive to set the stage for the period of the Renaissance and produced at least five major accomplishments. These achievements were:

1. Conversion of the invading barbarians.
2. Constriction of Islamic empire.
3. Extension of Christianity to the north and east.
4. Establishment of universities.
5. Creation of a complex network of new commercial centers and trade routes.

*I dressed him and God healed him.*—AMBROISE PARÉ

*Anatomy brought life and liberty to the art of healing, and for three centuries the great names of medicine were those of the great anatomists.* —SIR WILLIAM OSLER

# XIII Medicine of the Renaissance

THE RENAISSANCE was a time of transition between medieval and modern and was characterized by the beginnings of the Reformation, new literature and learned studies and great geographical discoveries. Various dates during the second half of the fifteenth century have been assigned to the origins of this period. These dates include:

1. 1453 (when Greek scholars migrated to the West because of the Fall of Constantinople),
2. 1454 (when printing was discovered), and
3. 1492 (when America was discovered).

The powerful rulers of Italian cities competed for scholars to translate classics from Greek to Latin. The work in literature and learned studies, known as Humanism, stressed the rebirth of the concept of the dignity of the individual and a desire for spiritual freedom. Biblical study merged into the religious movement of the Protestant Reformation which began in Germany in 1517 and the Catholic Reformation which was furthered by the founding of the Jesuit Order in 1540. The Renaissance period of medicine has been dated to the discovery of the work of Celsus in 1443 and the printing of his works in 1478.

Two new and pressing problems involved the attention of physicians and surgeons during the early period of the Renaissance, i.e., gunshot wounds and syphilis.

## GUNSHOT WOUNDS

It is believed that firearms and cannon were invented in the thirteenth century. They not only revolutionized warfare but introduced a new era of surgery. Cannon are said to have been employed at the seige of Metz in 1324. The importance of firearms and cannon as weapons of war came mainly with the battles of Ravenna (1512), Marignano (1515) and Pavia (1525). The problems of wound infections and of amputations became exceedingly common and no textbook on surgery was complete without a treatise on gunshot wounds.

## SYPHILIS

Syphilis appeared near the end of the fifteenth century in epidemic form. There is still controversy regarding the origin of the disease with two schools of thought prevailing. Sudhoff and his school of historians believed that the condition was prevalent in Europe for a long period of time previously. Others believed that it was brought to Europe by the sailors of Columbus following their return from America. Syphilis has been called "the epidemic of the fifteenth century." It spread to France, Germany, Switzerland, Holland, Greece, England, Scotland, Hungary and Russia, in that order, and was probably facilitated by public baths which had to be closed because of the epidemic. Most physicians blamed venereal contact as the cause. Some theologians and physicians saw the disease as a "plague sent down from Heaven." Astrologers said that it "took the beginning from Saturn when he entered into Aries." The French called it the disease of Naples and the Neopolitans called it the French disease. It was commonly called Morbus Gallicus (French Disease) until 1530 when the term *syphilis* was introduced by Girolamo Fracastoro. His famous poem described the legend of a shepherd known as Syphilis who was struck with the French disease because of an act of impiety.

Fracastoro's work on infection was his most original medical contribution and was published in 1546. This writing contains the first scientific statement of the true nature of contagion, of infection, of disease germs and of the modes of transmission of various diseases. He was ahead of his time and his ideas were obliged to await the discovery of the microscope.

Other physicians of the early Renaissance era made important contributions to the changing times. Some of these men were Antonio Benivieni, Giovanni di Vigo, Nicolo Leoniceno, Gerolamo Cardano, Gaspare Talliocozzi and Philip Theophrastus (Paracelsus).

## EARLY RENAISSANCE MEN

Antonio Benivieni (1443–1502) published the first book on pathological anatomy in 1507 in Florence. This was a collection chosen from his case records and edited soon after his death by a Florentine physician, Giovanni Rosati, at the request of Benivieni's brother, Geronimo. His title was *De abditis morborum causis* [The Hidden Causes of Diseases] and was the first report in modern literature of postmortem examinations made specifically to find out the cause of death. Others were slow to follow but he blazed a path for the work of Bonetus (172 years later) and for Morgagni (254 years later).

Giovanni di Vigo's *Practice of Surgery* was completed in 1513, was translated widely and became the authority on surgery during the sixteenth century. He accepted cauterization of wounds as the standard practice of the day. He made no significant new contributions. Di Vigo came to Rome in 1503 and became surgeon to Pope Julius II and had considerable service in his armies. This was the generation which also included Bramante who was erecting Saint Peter's Church, Michelangelo who was painting the ceiling of the Sistine Chapel in the Vatican and of Raphael who was creating his frescoes on the walls of the Vatican.

Nicolo Leoniceno was a Greek scholar and humanist. His major publication in 1492 concerned the errors of Pliny. He was also a critic of Avicenna and of the Arabic School.

Gerolamo Cardano gave the first clear

account of typhus fever in 1536. He was a graduate of Padua and because of difficulty in becoming admitted in the college of physicians in Milan, reacted with a book that contained a castigation of the poor medical practices of his colleagues and also an account of typhus fever. By 1552 he was commonly regarded as one of the greatest physicians and scholars in Europe.

Gaspare Talliocozzi published a classic in the history of plastic surgery in 1597. Talliocozzi was a Bolognese surgeon. His text described operations for the restoration of lost noses, lips and ears and included the story of rhinoplasty.

Philip Theophrastus (Paracelsus) (1493–1541) was born in Switzerland and has been called the "Luther of Medicine" by his admirers (Fig. 19). He wrote on alchemy, astrology, the occult arts and medicine. He considered the four pillars of medicine to be philosophy, astrology, alchemy and virtue. He broke with the accepted theory of disease (the humoral theory of Galen) and declared that health depended upon five active principles: stars, poisons, nature of the individual, influence on the spirit and the will of God. His work on syphilis was excellent and he wrote the first comprehensive account of an occupational disease (Miner's Disease). His work on mental disease was classic. Although his emphasis on chemistry in medicine was not original, it was a considerable contribution and his assault on Galen and on herbal polypharmacy stimulated controversy and investigation. He further upset tradition by lecturing in German (not Latin). He publicly burned Avicenna's *Canon* in order to symbolize his break with his colleagues on the faculty of the University of Basel. He wandered from city to city over a period of thirteen years. He was a heretic but did stimulate controversy and change.

The scholarly and humanistic spirit of antiquity guided the early Renaissance, and it was at first largely secular and religiously tolerant or skeptical. The Reformation was devoutly religious, often intolerant, frequently superstitious, harsher, more active and preoccupied with the future.

The artistic movement of the Renaissance in Italy was also carried into science. Some of these remarkable artists began anatomical dissection in order to improve upon the knowledge of the Greek artists whose knowledge was limited to the appearance of the outside of the body.

Leonardo da Vinci (1452–1519) was one of the artists who became adept at dissection. His collaborator was Marcantonio della Torre who began a comprehensive work on anatomy in Pavia but, unfortunately, died at the age of thirty-three before completing his work. Da Vinci made extremely accurate drawings. Seven-hundred and fifty separate anatomical sketches have been accumulated from his manuscripts. He is generally believed to have been the most versatile genius of the Renaissance and the most remarkable mind of history. Following his death, there was a lag in the history of anatomy for a generation.

## THE RENAISSANCE AND THE RISE OF ANATOMY

Anatomy, like all sciences, had its roots in the past. Herophilus (about 300 B.C.) was the first to practice dissection of human and animal bodies, according to Galen. Singer surmises that this means that he was the first to do so in public. From that time on, anatomical knowledge was based largely on animal dissection because

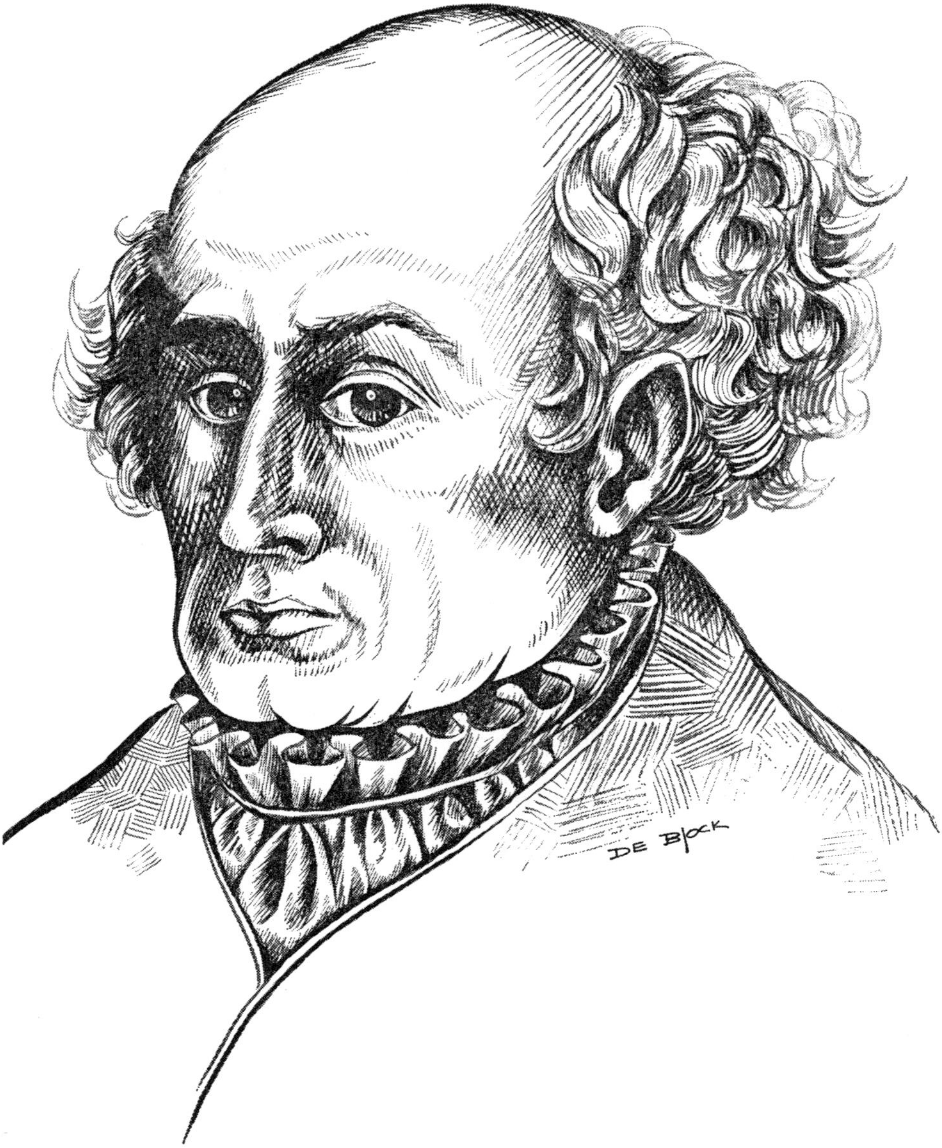


FIGURE 19. Paracelsus

human dissection was illegal during the Roman period and forbidden to Islamic physicians. There are, however, hints in the writings of Galen that suggest that he did dissect the human body. He constantly states that human dissection is the most desirable and that the ape is the next best. Galen's public dissections in Rome were usually carried out on apes or lower animals. As physician to the Emperor Marcus Aurelius he obviously did not court disfavor by doing otherwise.

William of Saliceto was said to have been the first to dissect the human body in Bologna. Mondino made the first public anatomical demonstrations in 1350 and started the famous School of Anatomy at the University of Bologna.

Artists played an important role in the early development of anatomy and the attendance of artists and sculptors at dissections was commonplace. The anatomical work of Leonardo da Vinci in connection with the dissections of della Torre has been mentioned. Albrecht Dürer published his *Human Proportions* in 1528 and was influenced by Leonardo. His work was that of an artist for artists rather than for physicians.

Berengario da Carpi (1470–1530) was the first to make comprehensive anatomical illustrations from nature. He graduated from Bologna, taught there at Pavia and practiced surgery in Rome and Ferrara. He is said to have dissected several hundred bodies. He followed the pattern of Mondino with his commentaries and also showed originality. He was the first to distinguish between lymphatic and venous structures, to describe the vermiform appendix, to give a clear account of the thymus gland and to describe a horse-shoe kidney. He discussed the action of the valves of the heart and is credited with the introduction of mercury in the treatment of syphilis.

Charles Estienne (1503–1564) was the last of the important anatomists prior to Vesalius. He was a member of a famous family of humanist printers and graduated from the University of Paris. His anatomy followed that of Galen and his illustrations were the earliest, except for Leonardo's, to show the whole arterial, venous and nervous systems. Many of his illustrations have been described as being horrible because they depicted the anatomy of criminals who had been beheaded for their crimes.

Andreas Vesalius (1514–1564) was the dominant figure in the field of anatomy in the Renaissance. His family showed a long devotion to the cult of Aesculapius for many generations. His classical education was completed at the University of Louvain and he entered formal medical education at the University of Paris in 1533. The university and its medical school were extremely conservative. Vesalius probably did not witness more than three or four anatomical demonstrations during his stay in Paris and knowledge of anatomy was necessarily gained largely from textbooks and the study of disarticulated bones. His teachers were largely loyal to Galen. His more important teachers were Günther of Andernach, Jacobus Sylvius and Jean Fernel. Vesalius accepted the Galenical anatomy like the other students of his time, but dissection and instruction at the dissection table was not available to him in Paris except on his own initiative. He acquired a considerable knowledge of anatomy by the dissection of animals and this led to his being requested by his teachers and fellow students to assist in demonstrations. He was obliged to leave Paris in 1536 after a period of three years because of the outbreak of war and the need for him as an imperial subject to return home. He was granted permission by the magistrates of Louvain to conduct "an anatomy" before eager fellow students. The ensuing year led to his thesis. It is assumed that a degree was granted by the University of Louvain but no record of his graduation in that institution is available. Seeking greater opportunities for the study of anatomy and medicine, he set out for the University of Padua, studied, and received the degree of doctor of medicine in December of 1537 "with highest distinction." He apparently made a profound impression on the faculty because he was almost immediately appointed as Professor of Surgery with responsibility to teach anatomy. He became friends with his countryman, Jan van Calcar, who was later to be associated with some of his publications. Van Calcar was, himself, new in Venice in order to study art in the school of Titian.

Vesalius' classes became crowded with students, physicians and men of learning and he introduced large charts to illustrate his views. He and van Calcar published six of these plates in 1530 without title. They are known as *Tabulae Anatomicae Sex* and represent his first anatomical publication. This was highly successful but many Galenical errors persisted. He continued to dissect and to lecture constantly during the next five years.

It is not known how long Vesalius had his composition of a major textbook of anatomy in mind. He was apparently deeply disturbed by discrepancies in the traditional teachings. It has been assumed that the composition of his text began in 1538. The publication of *De Humani Corporis Fabrica* [On the Fabric of the Human Body] in 1543 marked the beginning of modern biological science. It is a magnificent blend of creative art, typography and illustration. Careful examination of the plates of the *Fabrica* suggest participation of several artists and possibly the school of Titian. The *Epitome* also appeared in 1543 and a second edition of the *Fabrica* appeared in 1555. The *Fabrica* is one of the landmarks in the history of man's progress. Its impact was felt throughout the medical world and upset much of what had been accepted for more than thirteen-hundred years after the death of Galen. Vesalius (Fig. 20) became court physician to Emperor Charles V in 1544 and spent the rest of his life at court or in wars with Charles and his armies.

Bartolomeo Eustachi (1520–1574) was Vesalius' contemporary in Rome. He had little influence on anatomy while alive, but the discovery of his unpublished copper plates in the eighteenth century raised him to almost the same plane as Vesalius. His work was probably more accurate, but less pleasing. The middle ear canal is known as the eustachian tube. This was described by him but actually was known to Alcmaeon in 500 B.C. Eustachi discovered the thoracic duct and did excellent work on the muscles of the face and larynx and on the sympathetic nervous system.

Vesalius was succeeded by a series of illustrious anatomists at Padua. Some of his successors were Colombo, Fallopio, Fabrizi, Casserio and Spiegel.

Realdo Colombo (1516–1559) discovered that blood passes from the lung into the pulmonary vein. This discovery of the lesser or pulmonary circulation was actually first discovered by Annafis of Damascus more than two-hundred years earlier and was also independently found by Michael Servetus in 1553. The work of Servetus was unknown until one-hundred and forty-four years later. Colombo placed the lens in its proper position in the eyeball correcting Vesalius who had placed it in the center of the eyeball.

Gabriele Fallopio (1523–1602) succeeded Colombo at Padua. His *Observationes Anatomicae* was published in 1561. He described Berenegario da Carpi as the first restorer of anatomy and Vesalius as its perfector. Fallopio described the tubules

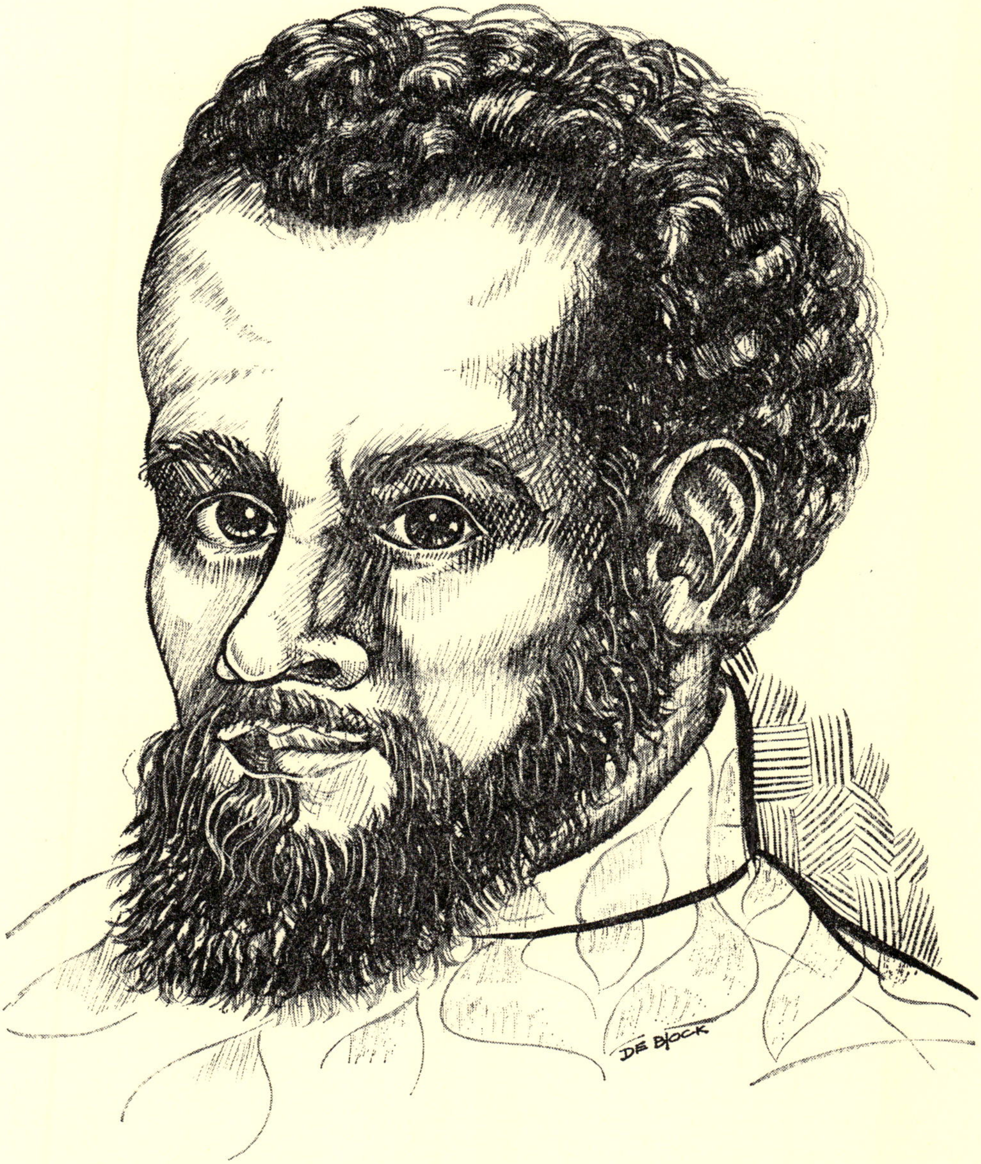


FIGURE 20. Andreas Vesalius—"Father of Anatomy."

from the ovary to the uterus, the chorda tympani, the semicircular canals, the sphenoidal sinuses, the aqueduct of Fallopius and he introduced the terms vagina, placenta, cochlea, labyrinth, palate and velum palati.

Girolamo Fabrizi (1537–1619) succeeded Fallopio. He was one of the greatest teachers of anatomy of all time and built an anatomical theater in Padua at his own expense for his students. This theater is still preserved but is not in use. Better known as Fabricius, he demonstrated and published on the valves of the veins and their functions in 1603. He made the first study of this kind in comparative embryology in animals and man and this magnificent work, *De Formato Foete,* remains a classic. His most famous pupil was William Harvey who based part of his later discovery of the circulation of blood upon Fabricius' study of the structure and functions of the veins.

The next anatomists at Padua were Casserio (1561–1616) and Spiegel (1578–1625). Spiegel was the last of the line of Vesalian anatomists of Padua. Spiegel described the lobe in the liver, now termed the *spiegelian lobe,* in his text, *De humani corporis fabrica,* which he published in 1627. By this time the best minds of medicine seemed to be drawn from the dissecting rooms to the new science of physiology and the Renaissance movement had spread to France and to Europe in general.

## FRANCE AND THE RENAISSANCE

Although King Charles VIII of France had failed to conquer Constantinople, his expedition marked the introduction of the Renaissance into France because of the relationships between Italy and France from 1494 to 1589. The introduction of Humanism and its spirit of free inquiry and human independence into France stimulated the growth of the Huguenot party and produced John Calvin who was one of the outstanding leaders of the Protestant revolt against the power of the Church. The scholars in turn, were accused by the Church of immorality, heresy and atheism. It tightened its hold on the University of Paris where scholasticism had held out successfully against the advance of Humanism for years. The other French seats of learning were affected in a similar manner.

During the fifteenth and sixteenth centuries, the medical profession in Paris was divided into three classes: (1) physicians; (2) surgeons, and (3) barber surgeons. Physicians were graduates of a school of medicine. They attempted to regulate surgical practice but did not operate themselves. Surgeons of the Confrerie (College) of St. Come wore long academic robes, treated wounds and abscesses, applied plasters and ointments, used cautery, but did not operate otherwise. Barber surgeons attempted many types of major surgery because of the needs of the military and their wounds. They shaved their customers and also practiced bloodletting (venous section) by cupping and leeching. In spite of these obstacles, some outstanding physicians and surgeons developed in France. Five of these more unusual individuals include: Sylvius, Fernel, De Baillou, Tagault and particularly Paré.

Jacobus Sylvius (1478–1555) was the Professor of Anatomy at the University of Paris. Among his illustrious pupils were Vesalius, Servetus and Estienne. Sylvius was regarded as the foremost anatomist of his period (prior to his pupils). His works were concise and well-written. He named a large number of muscles and blood vessels with names that they still bear. The aqueduct between the third and fourth ventricles of the brain was named for Sylvius. His respect for Galen and classical antiquity was such that he became estranged from his most famous pupil, Vesalius, whose original work was instrumental in creating the Renaissance of medicine.

Jean Fernel (1497–1558) was probably the outstanding physician of this period in

France. He was a member of the faculty of the University of Paris, a humanist, scholar and was consumed with a burning desire to extend the bounds of human knowledge. He was famous as a physician throughout Europe and was respected and loved by his students. He was hostile to the current beliefs in astrology and bloodletting. His teachings and great ability created an atmosphere of hostility and envy by most of his colleagues. He published a text in 1542 known as *On The Natural Part of Medicine.* Fernel was probably the first to describe the central canal of the spinal cord and he made many original physiological observations in the field of peristalsis and in the increase of the size of arteries during systole. He also published work on pathology and on venereal disease.

Gauillaume de Baillou (1538–1616) was the first modern epidemiologist. He provided excellent descriptions of plague, diphtheria, rheumatic fever and the earliest clear account of whooping cough.

Jean Tagault's text, *On Surgery,* was published in 1543 and was derived mainly from Guy de Chauliac and other previous authorities. It was written in Latin and was popular.

Ambroise Paré was the towering surgical figure of this period (Fig. 21). He was born in 1510 and lived to be eighty years of age. He was twelve years younger than Fernel and twenty-seven years older than Baillou. He was of extremely humble origin and started as a barber-surgeon in Paris. Soon after coming to Paris, Paré became a house officer in the Hôtel Dieu. He remained for a period of four years in this hospital which was not only the oldest in continuous service (founded 1443) but was also the largest in Paris. He spent most of his life going to war. Between wars he returned to Paris and was attached to various officers and finally to King Henry II. He was urged by Jacobus Sylvius to record his experiences on the treatment of war wounds. His books were all in French because he knew no other language. In that they were translated widely, created some controversy and had merit, his fame was established. His text, *On Gunshot Wounds,* was published in 1545 and did much to stop the current use of burning oil in wounds. He was received into the Confrerie of St. Come in 1554 and was given a degree of master of surgery. King Henry II sustained a severe head injury during a joust in 1559. He was attended by both Ambroise Paré and Andreas Vesalius. He died eleven days after his injury. The cause of death was probably a chronic subdural hematoma. The nature and surgical treatment of this condition was to be obscured until nearly three-hundred and sixty-six years later.

Paré's publication, *On Surgery,* was highly critical of the use of cautery in surgery and described the use of ligatures in amputations. Henry II was succeeded by Charles IX who persecuted the Huguenots. The new king was responsible for the massacre of St. Bartholomew in 1572 at which time two-thousand Huguenots were slain in Paris. It is stated that he wished to kill all Huguenots "except Master Ambroise Paré" who was his first surgeon. In the year of the massacre, Paré published another book containing entirely new material and forming one of his most important contributions to surgical literature. It dealt chiefly with the science of fractures and dislocations, gave current teaching about bandages and contained the first descrip-

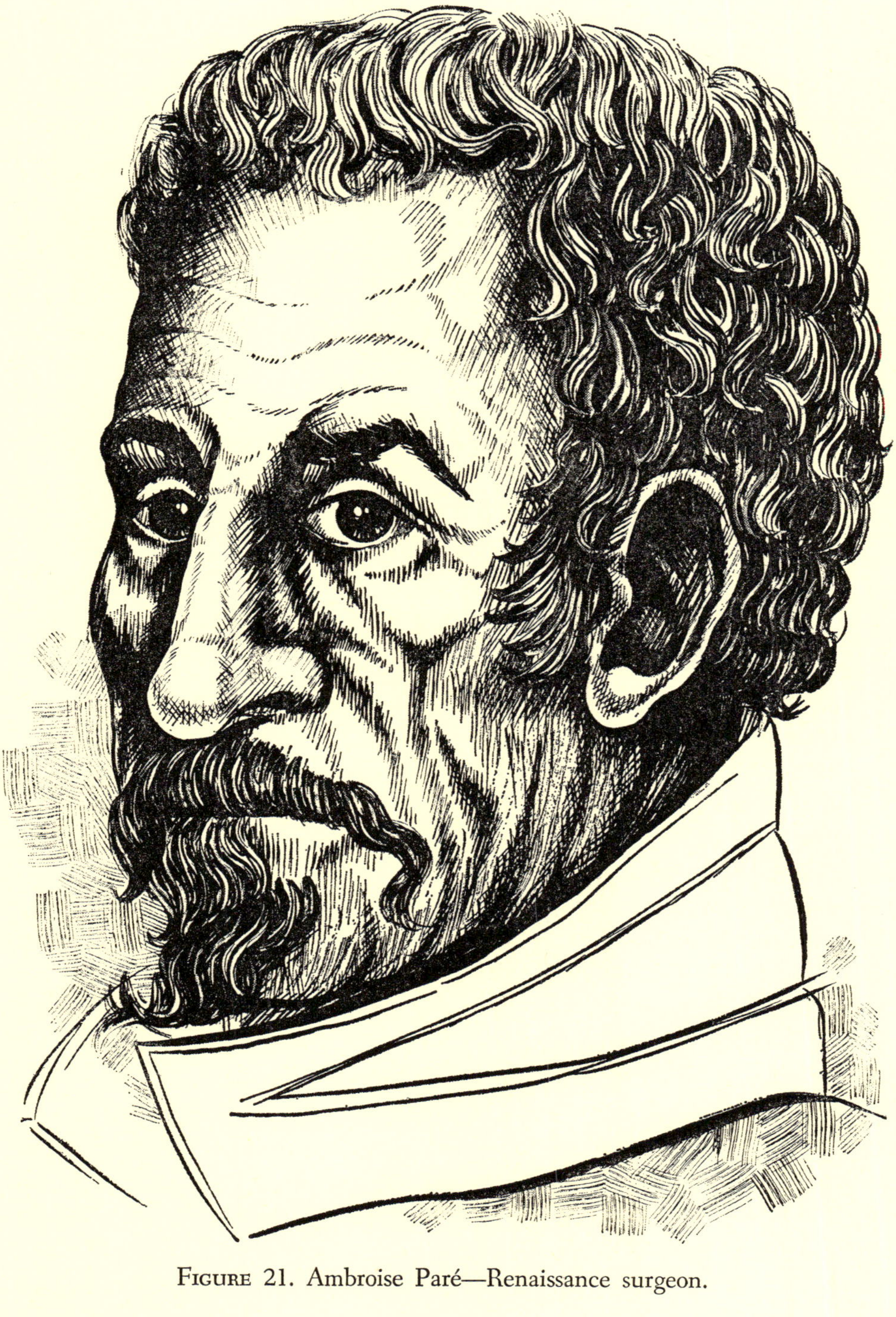

FIGURE 21. Ambroise Paré—Renaissance surgeon.

tion of fracture of the head of the femur. King Charles IX died in 1574 and was succeeded by his brother Henry III who kept Paré in his service. In 1575 Paré published the first edition of his *Oeuvres*. This book soon took its place as one of the most enlightened works on surgery ever published and placed the two sciences of medicine and surgery in their proper relationship and emphasized superiority of independent observation over blind acceptance of dogma. This splendid surgical treatise was as important in its sphere as the *Fabrica* of Vesalius was in anatomy thirty years earlier. There was no comparable surgeon during his time in any other country. His contributions included the emancipation of surgery from the dead hand of dogma, the harmfulness of treating gunshot wounds with boiling oil, the use of the ligature in amputation, and the podalic version in obstetrics.

## GERMANY AND THE RENAISSANCE

The Renaissance movement in Germany was feeble in comparison to Italy or France in relation to its impact on medicine. This is probably due to the small number of German universities and the fact that the ambitious young German who wished to study medicine went to Italy if he could afford to do so. The medical faculties of the German universities usually had only one or two professors and a correspondingly small number of students. This situation existed for several centuries after they were founded. The oldest German university was located in Prague in 1347. The next two universities to be founded in Germany were those in Heidelberg (1386) and in Leipzig (1409). Nevertheless, some major medical contributions were made during this period by a few German individuals, including von Pfolspeundt, Braunschweig, von Gerssdorff, Rosslin, Platter, Bartisch and Fabry.

Heinrich von Pfolspeundt was a member of the order of Teutonic Knights. He learned surgery mainly from warfare and from barber surgeons. Like other surgeons of the fifteenth century he was generally regarded in a low class of society. He was one of the earliest surgeons, if not the first, to describe gunshot wounds and to mention the extraction of bullets. He advised cutting both ends around an injury of the intestine and to unite them with silk over a silver tube. This was a precursor of the "Murphy Button" of 1892. He wrote a German text on surgery in 1460.

Braunschweig was a well-educated surgeon in Strassburg where surgeons were regarded as belonging to a learned profession. He published the first German manual of surgery in 1497 and this was translated into English and published in 1525. This was the first illustrated work on surgery in the English language.

Hans von Gerssdorff published his text on surgery in 1517 and this contained the first-known illustration of an amputation.

Eucharius Rosslin published the first separate work on obstetrics in 1513. This text, the *Rosegarten,* was small, popular and went through 100 editions. It marked the beginning of the renaissance of obstetrics. It was for pregnant women and midwives and was done in German. At this time, midwives monopolized the practice of obstetrics. The text contained twenty woodcuts and illustrated a birth chair, lying-in room, and positions of the foetus *in utero*. It was largely a compilation of writers on obstetrics from Hippocrates to Savonarola and especially Soranus and the work of a medieval translator by the name of Muscio.

Felix Platter was the first to carry out dissection of the human body in any Germanic country and was one of the earliest champions of Vesalius. He began his work in 1557 and published texts on anatomy, wrote excellent descriptions on myxedema and gall stones, and was the first to describe a persistent thymus gland and thymic death.

Georg Bartisch published the first German text on ophthalmology. His *Augendienst* was printed in 1583 and showed some familiarity with medical literature. He was born in 1535 at Konigsbruck. He later traveled with barbers, stonecutters, tooth pullers, charlatans and learned what he could of the healing arts. He continued his life as an itinerant surgeon even after he was appointed as court oculist by the Duke of Saxony. His trips were announced by leaflets which were distributed in the towns he planned to visit. These tracts extolled his skill in the curing of toothaches, stones of the bladder, removal of cataracts, et cetera, "with the help of God."

Wilhelm Fabry of Hilden (1560–1634) has been called the "Father of German Surgery." He received a classical education at Cologne. He was obliged, because of the death of his father, to apprentice himself to a barber surgeon with whom he served for four years. As the first educated and scientific German surgeon, he fought superstitions, irrational methods and spoke against witches and condemned torture. He made many dissections, taught anatomy and authored twenty medical books. He was probably the first to recommend amputation above the diseased part of problems of gangrene. He was also probably the first in western Europe to apply the magnet for the extraction of an iron splinter from the eye. The magnet had been used previously for the removal of iron splinters from the body by Susruta and by Ibn al-Tilmidh. Fabry is credited with being the first to recognize a case of congenital pyloric stenosis.

## ENGLAND AND THE RENAISSANCE MOVEMENT

The Renaissance movement did not affect England much at first because of her insular position. However, many young Englishmen studied in the Italian universities and returned to England to transplant this new learning to the homeland. Outstanding among these men at this time were John of Arderne, Thomas Linacre, Thomas Vicary and John Caius.

John of Arderne has been called the "Father of English Surgery." He was born in 1307, was well educated, wrote in Latin and served as an army surgeon in the Hundred Years' War with France during part of his career. He taught that wounds should heal without suppuration, that wounds should not be covered with irritating solutions, that dressings should be changed infrequently and that a fistula *in ano* should be divided from end to end. His operation for fistula *in ano* fell into disuse but has been universally employed during the past five hundred years.

Thomas Linacre (1460–1524) was educated in Italy and obtained his medical training at Padua. He then settled in Oxford where he taught Greek and practiced medicine. He was a scholar and a skillful physician. He translated Galen from Greek to Latin and was a powerful force in the spread of Humanism in England. It was his idea to establish the Royal College of Physicians in London. This organization was chartered by King Henry VIII, in 1518. Linacre was its first president with the power to examine and to license candidates to practice medicine.

The status of surgery and of surgeons in England closely resembled that of France at this time. Surgery was subordinate to medicine and remained in this state until our own times.

The Military Guild of Surgeons was formed in 1369. Army surgeons, who were serving individual commanders, formed this society. They required their members to have an apprenticeship for six years and then an examination by the masters of the guild prior to membership. If they failed the examination, they were obliged to serve another six years of apprenticeship. They were required to leave the field of surgery if they failed a second time.

The Guild of Barber Surgeons was formed in 1300. British barber surgeons formed this guild just as there were organizations for weavers, goldsmiths and merchants. Each guild member had a distinctive garb, according to his vocation. The apprentices of the Guild of Barber Surgeons received lectures, dissections, demonstrations and were licensed to practice in the city where the guild had its seat. These guilds became legal corporations which included all the British surgeons for a period of four hundred years. In 1313, an Act required everyone to belong to some guild and if the membership list in his own craft was filled, the individual must join another. Barber surgeons were frequently found in the guilds of silk weavers, cap makers, et cetera. The Guild of Barber Surgeons was incorporated in 1462 and then became known as a Company. It grew rapidly and became the largest of all the guilds with thirty-nine companies.

An Act of Parliament in 1511 also granted to the bishops the power to license practitioners and to punish offenders. The Royal College of Physicians was chartered in 1518 by another Act of Parliament at the instigation of King Henry VIII's physician, Linacre, and received the power to examine and license candidates.

Another Act of Parliament, in 1540, united the two surgical guilds (The Guild of Military Surgeons and the Company of Barber Surgeons) into the United Company of Barbers and of Surgeons. This Act specified that the surgeons were not to barber and the barbers were not to do surgery. It also provided bodies of criminals put to death for felonies for "anatomies" for members of the Company.

Thus, the official bodies which examined and licensed physicians and surgeons in England during the Renaissance were the universities, the bishops, the Royal College of Physicians, the Guild of Military Surgeons and the Company of Barber Surgeons until 1540 when the latter two groups were combined as the United Company of Barbers and of Surgeons.

Thomas Vicary was elected Master of the United Company of Barbers and of Surgeons at the time he was also surgeon to King Henry VIII. He was probably the Reader of Anatomy for the Company and wrote his unremarkable book in 1548.

John Caius succeeded Thomas Vicary. Caius was born in 1510, graduated from medical school in Padua and practiced in

Cambridge, Norwich and Shrewsbury. He had been a student of Vesalius and Colombo and remained as Reader in Anatomy for the Company of Barbers and of Surgeons for a period of twenty years beginning in 1543. He was a persistent Galenist and also became President of the Royal College of Physicians in 1555. He became physician to King Edward VI, Queen Mary and Queen Elizabeth, but was later dismissed by Elizabeth because of his adherence to the Roman Catholic faith.

## SUMMARY OF ADVANCES IN MEDICINE DURING THE RENAISSANCE

During the Renaissance period, medical thought changed rapidly. The rigid systems of Galen and Aristotle were replaced by Neoplatonism and objectivity of observations and experiments. The study of anatomy as part of observation of nature was one of the important gifts of the spirit of Humanism. The abandonment of the exclusive study of textbooks and the return to the study of the human organism and its behavior and diseases as an integral part of medicine, supplemented by information in textbooks was another significant contribution. Surgery made noteworthy progress in close connection with the new anatomical discoveries. New concepts in the field of epidemic diseases were introduced, particularly in relation to syphilis. Thus, the period of the Renaissance marked the return of the ancient Greek concepts in art, philosophy, literature and in medicine and a new science was founded on the basis of free, critical and individualistic studies.

*Genius is one percent inspiration and ninety-nine percent perspiration.*—THOMAS A. EDISON

# XIV Medicine of the Seventeenth Century

THE SEVENTEENTH CENTURY had no distinctive name such as did the fifteenth and sixteenth centuries (the Renaissance) and the eighteenth century (the Age of Enlightenment) but was fundamentally the most creative of the three periods.

From the viewpoint of world history, the greatest achievement of the seventeenth century was the development of modern science. This scientific revolution replaced previous concepts with new ideas of matter and its properties, new applications of mathematics to physics, and new methods of experimentation. By 1700, a "new world" view had taken form. Modern science rested on interchange and mutual verification of scientific ideas and information by investigators in many countries and these needs were satisfied by the development of scientific societies and publications. Scientific academies combined scientific and literary interests. Some were predominantly scientific such as the Lynxes of Rome (1603) and others were exclusively scientific such as the English Royal Society and the French Academy of Sciences founded in the 1600's.

The seventeenth century was also an age of religion, both Protestant and Catholic. Religion inspired the paintings of Rembrandt, El Greco, and many other outstanding artists. It also inspired the writings of Pascal in France, of Suarez in Spain and John Milton in England. Modern languages were perfected to convey exact and finer shades of feeling.

Italy no longer enjoyed its primacy and the center of gravity now shifted to northern Europe, southern England and Holland. London and Paris became the intellectual and cultural capitals of Europe.

The seventeenth century saw the decline of the Hapsburg supremacy, the rise of France on the international scene, the continuing disorganization of Germany, the development of monarchy in France and of constitutional government in England. The Thirty Years' War (1618–1648) represented conflicts between Catholics and Protestants in the major countries of Europe.

Two philosophers profoundly influenced the seventeenth century and also had an effect on its medicine. They were Bacon and Descartes.

Francis Bacon (1561–1626) was of the opinion that both philosophy and science must establish close relations between man and nature. He was a philosopher, lawyer, statesman, essayist and Lord Chancellor of England. He decried speculation about divine things or about the ultimate nature of things. He showed the vices of the scholastic method of the past and the sterility of tradition and dogmaticism in science. He brought out the faults of the Aristotelian system of syllogisms (reasoning from the general to the particular—deductive reasoning). He felt that anything worthy of belief should be capable of proof or demonstration. Science has never followed the method of Bacon completely, possibly because the number of facts is almost infinite, and personal or group judgment is necessary to select the pertinent facts. He developed inductive reasoning which is reasoning from the part to the whole, from the individual to the universal. His writings are given credit for being the impetus for the starting of the Royal Society.

René Descartes (1596–1650) devoted his entire life to scholarship in the fields of mathematics and philosophy. He invented analytical geometry and the statement of geometrical relationships in algebraic terms. He formulated the theory of "I think, therefore, I am." He was a major contributor to the modern theory of momentum, an explorer in the optics of vision, the proposer of an understandable dynamic theory of the mechanism of mind (or soul) and the inventor, in a rough way, of reflex action. He taught that all things in nature, animals and man, are machines which are composed of substances in movement. Descartes believed that an intelligent soul was located in the pineal gland of the brain and that the soul caused movement in the body by stirring up the brain, thus generating animal spirits in the cerebral ventricles with the spread of these spirits to cause movement of blood. His *Tractatus de homine* was published in 1662 and has been described as the first modern textbook of physiology.

Bacon, Descartes and all the earlier apostles of scientific reform made the mistake of imagining that a complete understanding of all events could be achieved within the period of a generation. The more modest Newton spoke of his efforts as a boy on the seashore picking up a few shells while the vast ocean of truth remained undiscovered. New discoveries in astronomy also had a powerful influence on philosophy, theology and science.

## THE BEGINNINGS OF ASTRONOMY

Pythagoras first proposed that the earth is a globe in the fifth century B.C. This was not confirmed until the Spanish crown had commissioned Ferdinand Magellan to seek out a new passage to the East and he circumnavigated the globe in 1519–1522.

Copernicus (1473–1543) a Polish medical graduate of Padua, studied astronomy in his spare time from medical practice in Frauenburg. He was influenced by Pythagoras, was not satisfied with the prevailing Ptolemiac concept of the universe and was convinced that the earth revolved about the sun. His theory was published in 1543.

Galileo was able to prove the correctness of Copernican theory by means of the use of the telescope which was invented in 1608 by Jansen. He published his work in his *Dialogue Concerning the Two Maximal Systems of the World* in 1632. He was imprisoned by the Inquisition because they thought that his views were not compatible with certain Scriptures. Although he was forced to deny his views and to do penance, his book was widely circulated and accepted in Europe.

Man and his world had suddenly become small in a very vast celestial system. It became apparent that Man and Earth were only small parts of a larger creation of God. These new discoveries in astronomy, therefore, had a powerful impact upon philosophy, theology and science. Other important developments related to medicine of the seventeenth century included the creation of instruments of precision and the rise of physiology.

## INSTRUMENTS OF PRECISION

Some of these instruments of precision were introduced into the practice of medicine by Santorio Santorio (1561–1636). He graduated from the school of medicine in Padua. He was physician to King Maximillian of Poland for fourteen years, professor at Padua for thirteen years and then practiced until his death in Venice. During his period of time in Poland he maintained close contact with both Galileo and Fabrizi of Padua. He was able to convert some of the brilliant ideas in the field of physics suggested to him by Galileo into practical measures which became valuable in clinical medicine. He made what was probably the earliest controlled study of basal metabolic rate (BMR). This work was published in 1614 and included a well-known illustration of the author seated in his steel yard chair about to weigh himself following a meal. He also weighed himself after a variety of activities. He weighed his food and his excreta and found that the weight of his excreta was less than the weight of his food. He reasoned that the food that he had ingested was not all excreted in feces, urine or invisible perspiration and that he must be exhaling part of the food stuff. He termed this method of exhalation as insensible perspiration. Santorio described and illustrated his pulsiolgium and thermometer in 1625 in Venice.

The microscope was another instrument of precision of first magnitude in the history of medicine. Apparently it was first invented about 1590 by Johannes Jansen and his son Zacharias. The Jansens were Holland spectacle makers. Their discovery spread through Italy. They also invented the telescope in 1608. Galileo constructed a microscope as well as a telescope as early as 1624.

The history of the microscope actually dates back to classical antiquity. Pliny mentioned the Roman use of both spherical and lens-shaped glasses for the purpose of burning as early as 77. Ibn al Haitham (935–1039) was an Arab physicist who described the magnifying power of the lens in his work on optics. Roger Bacon (1214–1292) described the lens for reading in these words: "useful to old men and those having feeble sight."

Salvino Armenti of Florence is believed to have invented spectacles. The use of spectacles and the manufacture of them spread over Europe and probably led to the invention of the microscope and telescope by the Jansens. (Armati died in 1317, some two-hundred and seventy-three years prior to the invention of the microscope.) This precision instrument was of interest only to the learned at first and it was a number of years before it was employed for medical studies. Four of the early microscopists were Kircher, Hooke, Malpighi and van Leeuwenhoek.

Athanasius Kircher (1602–1680) published a work in 1646 which included a chapter on "The Wonderful Structure of Things in Nature, Investigated by the Microscope" and the first-known illustration of the magic lantern and a great variety of other subjects. He published *Physico-Medical Scrutiny of the Contagious Pestilence* in 1658. This was certainly the first clear statement on the "germ theory" of contagious diseases based upon microscopical studies. Whether he actually saw the plague bacillus is open to question. Unfortunately, he was known to be a mystic and was superstitious and fond of bizarre speculations. It will be remembered that Fracastoro had written about the seeds of infection in 1546 prior to the invention of the microscope.

Robert Hooke (1635–1702) published *Micrographia* in 1665 and showed the histology of vegetable structures. He was apparently the first writer to employ the term *cell.* He also stated that the first microscopic drawings with which he was familiar were those of the London architect and Oxford physiologist, Christopher Wren. Hooke himself will be discussed later among the Oxford physiologists.

Marcello Malpighi (1628–1694) became Professor of Medicine at Bologna in 1656. He spent three years at the University of Pisa where he collaborated with Borelli and then went to Messina and finally returned to Bologna where he worked for the next twenty-five years. His *Anatomical Observations on the Lungs* in 1661 showed that the lung is made of numerous air vesicles in which the bronchioles end, and that a capillary anastomosis exists between the small arteries and veins. This came thirty-three years after William Harvey's discovery of the circulation of blood and provided the final needed anatomical link of evidence. Malpighi's *De formatione pulli in ovo* was published in 1666 and brought the previous work of Aristotle, Fabrizi, and Harvey to such perfection by using microscopical study that Malpighi has been called the "Father of Embryology." He also published on plant morphology and stressed the essential identity of plant and animal life.

Anton van Leeuwenhoek was born in 1633 in Holland. He understood only Dutch, ran a small dry-goods store and used his spare time to grind lenses, to make microscopes and to study objects with his microscopes. He described his observations with great accuracy and left speculation about interpretations to others. Among his friends and admirers was Reinier de Graaf, Delft's famous physician. De Graaf wrote to the Royal Society about Leeuwenhoek's investigations and this led to some two-hundred letters from Leeuwenhoek about his microscopic investigations to the Society and his election to its membership. These letters were translated into Latin or English and he became internationally famous. He described a large number of bacteria and protozoa. He suggested no relationship between these organisms and diseases. No one doubted that Leeuwenhoek saw the structures that he illustrated. He was visited by scientists from many lands. He has been described as the "Father of Protozoology and Bacteriology."

## THE RISE OF PHYSIOLOGY IN THE SEVENTEENTH CENTURY

The demonstration of the circulation of blood by William Harvey in his *De Motu Cordis,* which was published in 1628, ranks with Vesalius' *Fabrica* as a milestone in the progress of medicine and gave much impetus to the rise and development of physiology in the seventeenth century.

## Precursors to the Discovery of the Circulation of Blood by William Harvey

Previous workers had gradually developed knowledge about the heart and its vessels but a complete understanding of the circulation and the experimental proof of circulation is Harvey's contribution and his alone.

Galen (130–200) had demonstrated that arteries carry blood and not air and that venous blood was darker than arterial. He considered that blood ebbed and flowed in the heart and vessels but he did not understand circulation. Galen's theory assumed that blood passed from the right ventricle to the left through small openings in the interventricular septum. He conceived of the vascular system (Fig. 15) in relation to the psychosoma as follows:

| | *Natural Soul* | *Vital Soul* | *Rational Soul* |
|---|---|---|---|
| *Function* | Appetite<br>Nourishment | Emotions<br>Body heat | Thought and will<br>Emotion and sensation |
| *Seat* | Liver | Heart | Psyche |
| *Mediated by* | Blood | Arteries | Brain and nerves |

Annafis (Ibn al Nafis) of Damascus was an Arabian physician of the thirteenth century who discovered that the interventricular septum had no pores. He documented this in his *Commentary on the Anatomy of Avicenna's Canon.* He also gave the first clear statement of the pulmonary or lesser circulation two centuries before Servetus or Colombo. He stated that the blood "rises in the pulmonary artery to the lungs—to be mixed with air and passed to the pulmonary vein in which it is transmitted to the left cavity of the heart." This work remained unknown to the western world for seven centuries.

Andreas Vesalius (1514–1563) could find no pores in the interventricular septum and was frankly skeptical of blood passing through pores in this septum. However, he advanced no theory of his own. This point was a major one in the estrangement between Vesalius and his professor, Sylvius, who maintained Galenical doctrines.

Michael Servetus (1509–1553) was a physician, theologian and lawyer. In his work, *The Restoration of Christianity* (published in France in 1553), he documented his beliefs about the need for church reform and a return to simple Christianity and also discussed the vital spirit. In the latter discussion, he clearly described the pulmonary or lesser circulation. It will be recalled that, according to Galen, the vital spirits were located in the heart and by ebb and flow in blood vessels functioned to provide body heat and the emotions. Servetus' doctrine was that the blood passed from the right ventricle to the left, not through the septum, but by being transmitted from the pulmonary artery to the pulmonary vein by a lengthened passage through the lungs in the course of which it was elaborated and became a crimson color. His work was buried and unnoticed for one hundred forty-four years. He was imprisoned by the Inquisition as a heretic. He managed to escape to Geneva, Switzerland and sought the protection of the Protestant leader of the Reformation, John Calvin. Calvin was apparently as shocked as the Catholics were by Servetus' views on the Holy Trinity and on the uselessness of infant baptism. This led to his arrest. He was publicly burned at the stake in 1553 in Geneva, Switzerland.

Realdo Colombo (1516–1559) clearly

described the pulmonary circulation in his only book. This appeared in 1559 following his death. Colombo was a pupil of Vesalius at Padua and taught anatomy in Rome where he was acquainted with Michelangelo. The latter did not carry through with his promise to illustrate Colombo's text on anatomy and, accordingly, this book has only a frontispiece for an illustration. The discovery of the pulmonary circulation is usually associated with the names of Servetus and Colombo because the work of Ibn al Nafis was unknown to the western world until recently.

André Cesalpino was the first medical author to use the term *circulation*. He did so in his publication, *Question of Peripatetics*, which was printed in Venice in 1571. He was a physician, scholar, eminent botanist and was fond of theological and philosophical disputes. He seemed to describe accurately the circulation of blood without having a clear idea of circulation and he attempted to reconcile his views with those of Aristotle. For example, Cesalpino stated:

> The circulation of the blood which takes place from the right ventricle to the left ventricle, in passing through the lungs, agrees quite exactly with the following facts, which are apparent from dissection. There are two vessels which end in the right ventricle, two in the left. One of the two is afferent and the other efferent. . . . The blood is conducted to the heart by veins [and] is carried by the arteries throughout the body. The veins are engorged below a ligature, not above. Those who bleed patients are familiar with this experiment.

But he then spoils accuracy with this statement:

> When we are awake, a large supply of blood and spirits is conveyed to the arteries and thence to the nerves. When we are asleep, however, the same heat is carried back to the heart not by the arteries but by the veins.

His contemporaries were unimpressed by Cesalpino's doctrines. Their importance was stressed later, after they had been rediscovered.

## WILLIAM HARVEY AND THE DISCOVERY OF THE CIRCULATION OF BLOOD

William Harvey (1578–1657) is justly celebrated as the discoverer of the circulation of blood (Fig. 22). By experiment he proved his theory whereas others had only theorized. Harvey's work introduced experimental physiology to his own and succeeding generations. This science had been dormant since the death of Galen.

Harvey's entrance into Caius College at Cambridge implied the choice of a medical career. He started his training in 1593 (the same year that Cesalpino published his *Questiones Medicae* and, incidentally, discussed pulmonary and systemic circulation) and he began his medical studies at Padua in 1598 at the time that Fabrizi had just erected a new anatomical theater. The professor was loved and respected for his learning, charity and skill and apparently Harvey became one of his favorite pupils. Other members of the faculty included Casserio, Galileo and Santorio. He received his diploma of doctor of physic at Padua, returned to England and received a doctorate in medicine from Cambridge in 1602. During the following year, Fabrizi published his *De Venarum Ostiolis* and James I succeeded Queen Elizabeth. In 1604, Harvey married the daughter of Doctor Lancelot Browne, the physician to James I. He was elected as a fellow of the Royal College of Physicians in 1607—the

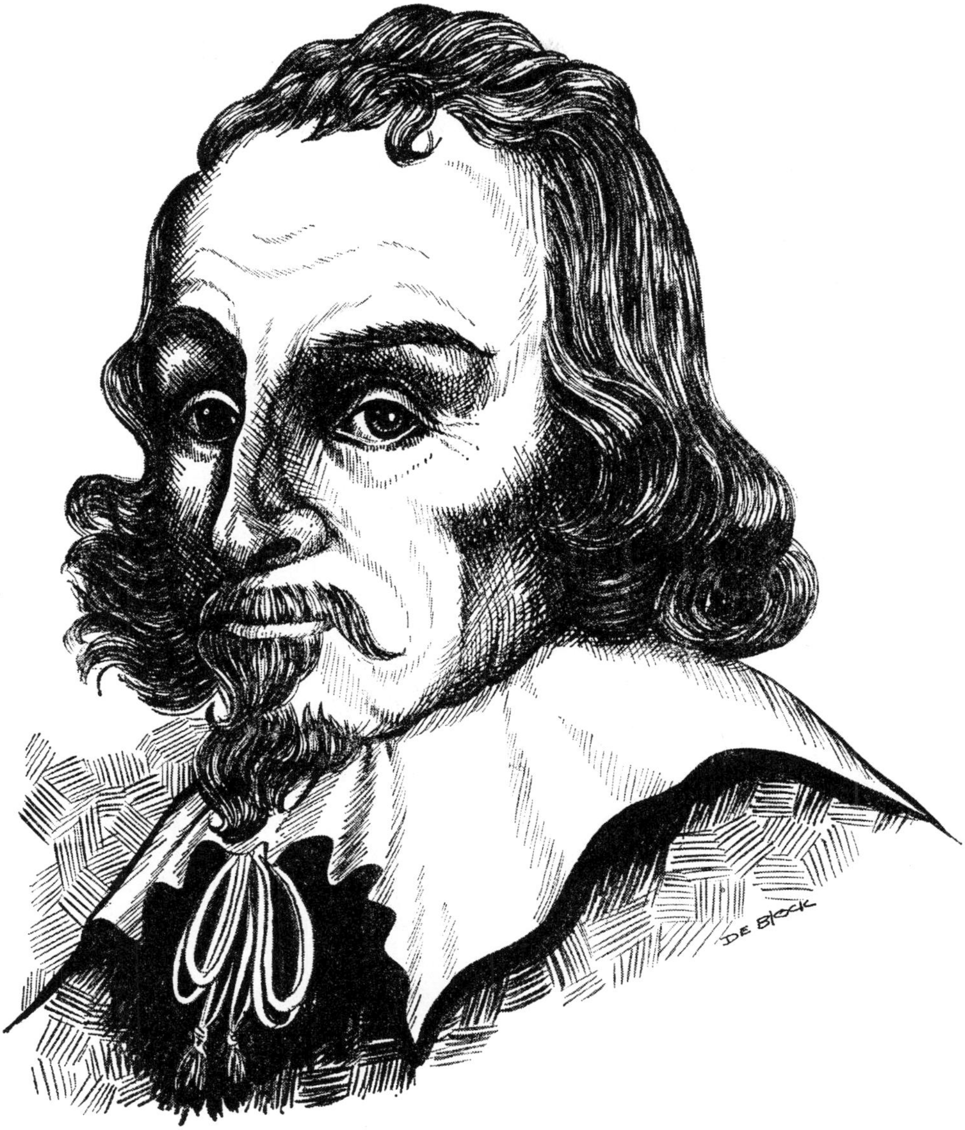


FIGURE 22. William Harvey—discoverer of the circulation of blood.

year that Jamestown, Virginia was settled.

The Lumleian Lecturer for the Royal College of Physicians on Surgery and Anatomy in 1616, was described as follows:

> William Harvey demonstrates by the structure of the heart that the blood is constantly passed through the lungs into the aorta . . . he demonstrates by the ligature, the passage of blood from arteries to veins. Thus, is proved a perpetual motion of the blood in a circle caused by the pulsation of the heart.

This is a summary of Harvey's views on the circulation of blood at this early date. He became the physician to James I and Francis Bacon, the Lord Chancellor, was his patient, but there was little sympathy between them. The Thirty Years' War began in 1618.

His masterpiece was *Exercitatio Anatomico de Motu Cordis et Sanguinis in animalibus,* commonly known as *De Motu Cordis.* This was published in 1628 at Frankfurt at the annual book fair, where a large circulation was hoped for. It is a model of Bacon's inductive reasoning and one of the most influential publications in medical history. The book, which was dedicated to King Charles I, began by emphasizing that it is necessary to observe the beating hearts of animals in order to understand circulation. Harvey then continued:

> When the left ventricle stops beating, the pulsations in the arteries cease. First the auricle contracts and this forces the abundant blood it contains . . . into the ventricle. This being filled, the heart raises itself, makes its fibers tense, contracts, and beats. By this beat, it at once ejects into the arteries the blood received from the auricle; the right ventricle sending its blood to the lungs through the vessel called the vena arteriosa (pulmonary artery) . . . the left ventricle sending blood to the aorta and to the rest of the body through the arteries.

He quoted the work of his old master, Fabrizi on the valves of the veins to reinforce his views that the veins carry blood to the heart, and agreed with "Colombo, the great anatomist, that blood passes from the right ventricle, through the lungs into the left auricle."

Robert Boyle asked Harvey how he came to think of the circulation of blood. Harvey replied,

> Since the blood could not well, because of the interposing valves, be sent by the veins to the limbs; it should be sent through the arteries and returned through the veins, whose valves did not oppose the course that way.

*De Motu Cordis* was received with varying reactions. It was ignored, battled and supported. Joannes Riolan, Professor of Anatomy at Paris, was the most determined opponent. John Aubrey in his *Brief Lives* wrote of Harvey as follows:

> I have heard him say that after his book on the Circulation of the Blood came out, that he fell mightily in his practice and twas believed by the vulgar that he was crackbrained; and all physicians were against his position and envied him. With much adoe, at least in about twenty or thirty years' time, it was received in all the universities in the world. . . . All his profession would allow him to be an excellent anatomist, but I never heard of any that admired his therapeutic way. I knew several practitioners in London that would not have given anything for one of his prescriptions.

He was appointed physician to Charles I in 1630 and drew up the rules governing Saint Bartholomew's Hospital in which he subordinated surgeons to physicians. He was ordered by Charles I in 1634 to examine the witches of Lancashire and was largely instrumental in obtaining their pardon from a death sentence. He was obliged to take charge of Prince Charles and Prince James when Charles I and his court fled London during the Civil War in 1642.

The significance of the revolution in medical thought brought about by Harvey's discovery increases with the years. The teaching of Galen had been regarded as infallible for fourteen hundred years and to depart from it was dangerous to reputation and sometimes even to life. Harvey's work showed how research should be done, and followed as much as possible the rules for the collection of facts and for inductive methods of thought advocated by Bacon. His methods, therefore, have since become a model for research; namely, careful observation, thoughtful deliberation, the appropriate experiment, and further consideration upon the results. His work provided the needed impetus to the development of physiology.

## PHYSIOLOGY IN THE SEVENTEENTH CENTURY

The physiology of the seventeenth century was developed along chemical or along physical and mechanical concepts.

The Iatrochemical School was that of a medical science based on chemistry. (*Iatro* is of Greek derivation and means physician, literally.) Johann Baptiste van Helmont (1577–1644) was the leading figure of this school of thought. He was born in Brussels just one year before the birth of Harvey. After studying medicine, philosophy and law at the University of Louvain, he practiced in Brussels until his marriage to an heiress. This enabled him to settle in nearby Vilvorde where he gave free medicine to the poor and spent the rest of his time with chemical observations and experiments. Ferments were the basis of his system of physiology. He stated that an acid ferment exists in the stomach but that the acid of the stomach is not, itself, the ferment. He found that the acid chyme in the stomach passes into the duodenum where it becomes alkaline and a second ferment is supplied by the bile. An American Army doctor elucidated the physiology of digestion two hundred years later. Van Helmont persisted in the Galenical beliefs regarding blood, vessels, ebb and flow of blood, et cetera. He described asthma vividly and correctly placed the trouble in the bronchi and attributed attacks of asthma to inhalation of house dust, ingestion of fish, et cetera. He introduced the terms *blas* (an invisible spiritual energy which governs all material changes) and *gas* (clearly carbon dioxide as produced by a ferment and not by air). Van Helmont was a dual personality. He was not only an excellent experimentalist who used sensitive balances and was able to devise a thermometer and to be the first to make gravimetric studies on the urine, but he was also a mystic and was very speculative. He believed in Paracelsus' weapon salve (healing by annointing the weapon instead of the wound) and magnetic and sympathetic healing. He was denounced for this by the Inquisition in 1624 and spent two years in prison.

The first chemical laboratory in a university was probably the one at the University of Leyden in Holland. This was built in 1658 for Franciscus Sylvius (no relation to the Parisian anatomist). This Sylvius was Professor of Medicine at Leyden. He studied acids, alkalies, salts, and explained many diseases on the basis of what we should today call acidosis and alkalosis. He introduced bedside teaching, stressed pathological studies, taught Harvey's doctrine of circulation and was interested in anatomy. He pointed out that the essential lesion in phthisis was the formation of tubercles in the lungs. He carried out many anatomical and physiological studies and was not the mystic that so many of those of his times were, including van Helmont. He was a fine teacher and students from all of Europe came to Leyden to work with him. Through his pupils he inspired much future investigation of importance but he himself made no great discoveries. Leyden later became the fountainhead of medical teaching and had a profound influence on the development of medicine in Vienna, Edinburgh, Europe, and America.

The Iatrophysical School was that of a medical science based on physics and mechanics.

Giovanni Alfonso Borelli (1608–1679) founded the iatrophysical school of thought which sought to prove that physiological conclusions could be developed from mathematics, physics and mechanics. Borelli became famous as Professor of Mathematics at the University of Messina and was called to a similar post at Pisa in 1656. He met Malpighi who had come to Pisa as Professor of Medicine the same year and became interested in his research and experiments. He divided movements into internal (heart, and viscera) and external (skeletal) investigating and describing them with the aid of mathematical calculations. He studied and clarified respiration, rejecting the age-old notion that respiration was for the purpose of cooling the innate heat of the heart and to expel the vapors caused by this heat. He clearly stated that inspiration was produced by the pressure and elasticity of the air, together with the increased size of the thorax brought about by muscular contractions and that expiration was the reverse. He was incorrect in giving a physical explanation and in rejecting the chemical hypothesis of the union of something in the air and the blood. His reasoning was clear, logical, and had a deep influence on the medicine of his time and upon his disciples. His *De motu animalium* appeared after his death in 1680–81.

## ENGLISH PHYSIOLOGISTS

The Royal Society in London and the Oxford physiologists played a significant role in the rise and development of seventeenth century physiology in medicine. The Royal Society actually began in about 1645 when a group of scientists formed a society which they called "The Invisible College." They met in their own lodgings or at Gresham College and when several of the members moved to Oxford their meetings were continued. Wars disrupted the activities of this group until the restoration of Charles II. They were reunited and organized with the approval of Charles II in 1660 as the Royal Society of London, with formal incorporation two years later.

Oxford University was more famous in the humanities at this time than in the natural sciences and received a new spirit from these young scholars in the Royal Society. Oxford physiologists included Boyle, Hooke, Wren, Lower, Mayow, Glisson and Willis.

Robert Boyle published his first book in 1660. This volume contained his Law: "At a stated temperature a given mass varies in a volume inversely to the pressure." He became associated with the Invisible College and was an incorporator of the Royal Society. He received his doctor of physic degree in 1665. Boyle advocated the atomic structure of matter in 1666 and shortly before his death stated the modern kinetic theory of gases (that a gas is a collection of free and independently moving molecules). He studied respiration, combustion, the chemical nature of blood and wine, magnetism, electricity and almost everything except for astronomy. He died in 1691.

Robert Hooke (1635–1702) was Boyle's pupil and was curator of the Royal Society until his death. His microscopic contributions have already been described. He performed his memorable experiment on artificial respiration in 1667 proving that the movement of the lungs was incidental to respiration and that the essential factor was the supply of fresh air. His experiment was to puncture the lungs in many places but to continue to pass air into them through the trachea. He found that although the lungs might be motionless, the heart would beat strongly as long as fresh air was supplied. Artificial respiration itself had been described one hundred twenty-four years previously in the last chapter of Vesalius' *Fabica.*

Christopher Wren (1632–1723) belonged to the Invisible College as an Oxford student. He assisted Thomas Willis in the preparation of his *Cerebri Anatome* which was published in 1664. He began his experiments with infusions in 1656. He injected wine, ale, opium and other substances into dogs intravenously and led the way for blood transfusions which were successfully performed for the first time in animals and man by Lower. Intravenous medications were first described by Johann Major at Kiel in 1664 and were suggested by the experiments of Wren. The latter also demonstrated that the removal of the spleen did not impair the health of the dog. After the great fire of London in 1666 he was appointed as the "Surveyor-General and Principal Architect for rebuilding the whole city, the Cathedral of St. Paul and all the parochial churches." His epitaph in St. Paul's Cathedral is *Si monumentum requiris, circumpice.*

Richard Lower (1631–1691) also assisted Thomas Willis on his memorable book, *Cerebri Anatome.* He successfully transfused the blood of one animal to another in 1665 and transfused a "poor and debauched man" with the blood of a sheep without complications in 1667. He published his *Tractatus de Corde* in 1669. This is a classic in medicine and contained the most accurate description of the anatomy of the heart to that date and one of the first examples of adherent pericardium. In addition, physiology of the heart and respiration and his method of transfusion were described.

John Mayow (1643–1679) believed that nitro-aerial particles were necessary to life. It was not until 1777 that Lavosier proposed the name "oxygen" and advanced the true meaning of this substance.

Francis Glisson (1597–1677) introduced a fundamental concept in the development of physiology in 1654, that of irritability as a property of living tissue. His monograph on rickets in 1650 was the first by an English author and it was he that called attention to Daniel Wistler's original article. His work, *De Hepate,* was published in 1654 and contained the best account of the anatomy of the liver up to that time. He described the sheath around the portal vein, hepatic artery and duct. This is now known as Glisson's capsule.

Thomas Willis (1621–1675) was the elder member of the Oxford group. When Willis was a medical student during the seige of Oxford, William Harvey was at that time Warden of Merton College and carrying out experiments in the vicinity. He turned his attention to "the Doctrine of the Nerves" and called this *neurology.* It was Willis, therefore, who originated the term for this specialty of medicine. He also wrote of "the Doctrine of the Brain." He published his *Cerebri Anatome* in 1664 and described the blood vessels at the base of the brain and their connections. These vessels are now known as the "circle of Willis." He also injected ink into the carotid arteries and showed that the fluid passed one way and then the other around this circle and ran on into the depths of the brain. This type of experimentation aided in the understanding of the physiology of the circulation of the brain and what would happen if one vessel should be closed. Richard Lower and Christopher Wren assisted him. Willis was also London's most distinguished physician. He was a keen observer and was the first physician in Europe to note the sweet taste of diabetic urine. He made classic descriptions of influenza, typhus and typhoid fevers, and noted the constriction of bronchioles in asthma. He also gave the earliest clearly obvious descriptions of hyperacusis, myasthenia gravis and cardiospasm. He was a follower of the iatrochemical school and speculated on fermentations.

## ANATOMICAL DISCOVERIES OF PHYSIOLOGICAL IMPORTANCE

The seventeenth century also brought many anatomical discoveries which had physiological importance. A partial list of these discoveries includes:

- Lacteal vessels—described in 1622 by Gasparo Aselli
- Lymphatic duct—described in 1651 by Pecquet
- Pancreatic duct—described in 1642 by Wirsung
- Maxillary antrum—described in 1651 by Highmore
- Submaxillary duct—described in 1656 by Wharton
- Haversian canals—described in 1691 by Havers
- Cowper's glands—described in 1694 by Cowper
- Pacchionian bodies—described in 1697 by Pacchioni
- Conjunctival glands—described in 1666 by Meibom
- Duodenal glands—described in 1682 by Brünner
- Graafian follicles—described in 1672 by de Graaf
- Parotid duct—described in 1662 by Stensen
- Lymphoid follicles in the intestine—described in 1677 by Peyer

## EPIDEMICS OF THE SEVENTEENTH CENTURY

Epidemics of plague and typhus continued into the seventeenth century. From 1618–1648 during the Thirty Years' War, Germany lost 50 to 75 percent of her population largely due to plague and typhus. The Venetian Republic lost more than five hundred thousand people because of plague in 1630. This epidemic swept over the Tyrol and the little village of Oberammergau. The village elders vowed that if God spared them, they and their descendents would do the Passion Play every ten years. London had its last great plague epidemic in 1665. It has been theorized that the great fire which destroyed London during the following year also eliminated plague infestation.

The list of eminent physicians of the seventeenth century is a long one.

## OTHER EMINENT PHYSICIANS OF THE SEVENTEENTH CENTURY

### England

English medicine of this period provided William Harvey, the Oxford physiologists, a superb anatomist-clinician, Thomas Willis, and also Sydenham and Wiseman, among other eminent men.

Thomas Sydenham (1624–1689) has been referred to as the "English Hippocrates." He was three years younger than Willis and had no sympathy for the anatomical and physiological experiments of the Invisible College. Unlike Harvey and Willis who were royalists, Sydenham fought in the Army of the Parliament against the King. He made slow progress in London and never became a Fellow of the Royal Society. He was not licensed to practice until 1667, after his fame had become established. He believed and taught that medicine could be learned only at the bedside. His descriptions of disease were unrivalled since the time of Hippocrates. He found that the Jesuit powder (quinine) was curative in fevers. He used quinine effectively, although many of his colleagues resisted this innovation.

Richard Wiseman (1622–1676) was admitted to the United Company of Barbers and Surgeons following a period of seven years as an apprentice and after service as a Dutch Navy surgeon through the war with Spain. He became Master of the Barber Surgeons' Company in 1665. His *Severall Chirugicall Treatises* was published in 1676 and represented a landmark in the history of British surgery. Wiseman represented a transition from the period when a surgeon learned from the school of warfare to a period when he saw his patients with a physician in civil practice and as a colleague.

## Holland

Holland became a great colonial power with a large empire in the distant East Indies during the seventeenth century. Bontius, Tulp and de Graaf were among the noted Dutch physicians of this period.

Jacob Bontius (1592–1631) graduated from the University of Leyden. He practiced for a period of four years in Batavia and Java and described tropical diseases, botany and fauna of the East Indies. He produced the first authoritative work on tropical diseases and the first description of beri-beri in the European literature.

Nicholas Tulp (1593–1674) was another distinguished Dutch physician. Rembrandt has immortalized Tulp dissecting before a group of doctors in his painting "The Anatomy Lesson." *Observationes Medicae* by Tulp was published in 1641 and included his description and illustration of the ileocecal valve (Tulp's valve) and indicated the follow-up of his diagnoses by postmortem examinations.

Reinier de Graaf (1641–1673) received his medical education at Utrecht and Leyden. While he was still a medical student in 1664, he published a treatise on pancreatic juice. He described and illustrated his method of collecting the juice through a cannula. He also obtained bile from the bile duct and saliva from the parotid gland by the same method. He published a volume containing three treatises in 1668 on the anatomy of the male and female organs of regeneration. The follicles of the ovary were described and have been called graafian follicles since that time. He thought these to be the egg but this error was corrected in 1826 by von Baer who showed the egg was actually within the follicle. This work also described clysters and discussed this popular therapy, the method of injection, and medicinals used and his syringe. De Graaf was Leeuwenhoek's friend and died at the age of thirty-two of plague, after practicing in Delft for about eight years.

### Switzerland

Theophile Bonet (1620–1689) graduated from Bologna and practiced medicine in Geneva, Switzerland until he became deaf at the age of fifty. He then spent the remainder of his life, a period of nineteen years, in studying and writing. He produced sixteen medical books. His first publication was the *Sepulchretum* in 1679. This ranks with the few medical books of importance and gave impetus to the study of pathological anatomy. He presented some three thousand protocols. Each was complete with clinical features and followed by their pathological findings and necropsy. This was an encyclopedia which contained a record of each recognizable disease from ancient times to that date. His work was influential in his time and was highly praised eighty years later by Morgagni who patterned his *De sedibus* after Bonet's work.

## SUMMARY OF THE CONTRIBUTIONS OF THE SEVENTEENTH CENTURY

During the seventeenth century, the advances made in medicine and in science during the Renaissance were consolidated. Philosophy and science were able to reestablish close relations between man and nature. Scholastic methods which had been dominant since the Middle Ages, dogmatism in science and the faults of the Aristotelian system of syllogisms were supplanted by advances in anatomy, chemistry, physiology, medicine and surgery. The demonstration of the circulation of blood by William Harvey was the outstanding scientific achievement of this century.

*When I was a boy I wanted to know about the clouds and the grasses, and why the leaves changed colour in the autumn; I watched the ants, bees, birds, tadpoles and cadis worms; I pestered people with questions about what nobody knew or cared about.*—John Hunter

# XV Medicine of the Eighteenth Century

The eighteenth century has been referred to as the Age of Enlightenment. Scientific, artistic and literary achievements of the seventeenth century were more widely projected in the eighteenth century both socially and geographically. This era seemed conscious of its intellectual emancipation and intent upon the benefits that might follow if new ideas were applied in practice.

London and Paris were the largest cities west of Constantinople and were the centers from which the majority of the ideas and institutions originated. In addition, scientific and literary academies of the type that had arisen from Italy to England during the preceding century were now established in Edinburgh, Dublin, Lisbon, Madrid, Berlin, Copenhagen, Stockholm, St. Petersburg and Philadelphia. A maritime England, a strong but not dominant France, a Danubian Austria, a westernized Russia, and Prussia and Savoy-Sardinia as kingdoms formed the nucleus of European powers which were to dominate European history for the next two hundred years.

France was looked to for cultural leadership and was greatly influenced by the parliamentary government and religious tolerance of England. French was the language of international relations, the second language of educated persons, the official language of the academies of Berlin and St. Petersburg until 1800 and this was carried into medicine.

The thought of the period was increasingly critical of aristocratic, monarchial and ecclesiastical institutions and led to a fifty-year period of revolution on both sides of the Atlantic Ocean, beginning with the American Revolution in 1776. The purpose and the ideals of the revolutionary movements in Europe and America were similar. Both desired political liberty, individual rights, national sovereignty, legal equality and a modern conception of law and citizenship with a State favorable to economic expansion and orderly government through written constitutions.

Newspapers and magazines became common. Museums were characteristic of the period and made scientific knowledge and works of art accessible to the public. The British Museum was founded in 1757 and the Louvre became fully opened after the French Revolution.

The eighteenth century has been described as an age of "Theorists and System-Makers" by the medical historian Garrison. Some followed the suggestion of Sydenham that the natural history of disease should be studied in the same spirit that natural objects were studied. Classifications of diseases into classes, orders and genera were developed because of this penchant. Philosophers became active in claiming that all knowledge was the domain of philosophy. The old schools of the iatrophysicists and iatrochemists were revived because of new discoveries in physics and chemistry. A fusion of these concepts with prevailing philosophical speculations was evident among some of the leaders in medical thought, particularly Stahl and Hoffmann.

George Stahl (1660–1734) was one of the leaders of this synthesis. He emphasized the unity of the living organism and combatted the one-sided materialism of his period. In his text, *Animism,* which was published in 1708 he expounded the theory that a supreme principle of life regulates all functions of the body during life but disappears at death. He called this principle the "anima" and disagreed with Descartes who distinguished sharply between the life of the soul and that of the body. He taught that fever was due to increased activity of the anima and should not be combatted in an attempt to restore health. He believed that if the anima was not successful in restoring health, the physician should assist with cathartics, venesection, emetics and methods to produce profuse sweating. He considered opium and quinine to be harmful to the anima. Stahl is remembered in chemistry as the promulgator of the phlogiston theory. Reminiscent of Jabir and first proposed by Becker, this theory held that combustible substances lose something when they are burned. The substance lost was called "phlogiston." This theory dominated chemical thinking until it was demolished by Lavoisier in 1777.

Freidrich Hoffmann (1660–1742) was a learned and kindly man. His chief work was his *Rational System of Medicine* which he published in nine volumes from 1718 to 1740. He taught that life is movement and that disease is due to spasm or atony. His therapy was simple, logical and counter to the prevalent polypharmacy of the time. He was one of the first to describe rubella and wrote excellent accounts of typhus fever and chlorosis. He originated Hoffmann's anodyne. Stahl and Hoffmann were Germans. Contemporary with these German leaders was a physician who added such luster to the University of Leyden in the Netherlands that this center developed the reputation that Padua had enjoyed two centuries previously (Fig. 23).

## THE UNIVERSITY OF LEYDEN

The history of Leyden goes back to about 1100 when a fortress developed. During the next several centuries, cloth-weavers and their industry made Leyden famous. However, the real fame of the city during the Renaissance period is associated with resistance by the population of Leyden under the leadership of William the Silent, Prince of Orange, against the Spanish beseiger, Valdez. As a reward, the old medieval industry city got the right to erect a university. The association of Bontius, Tulp, and Reinier de Graaf with Leyden in the seventeenth century has already been discussed. Herman Boerhaave (Fig. 24)

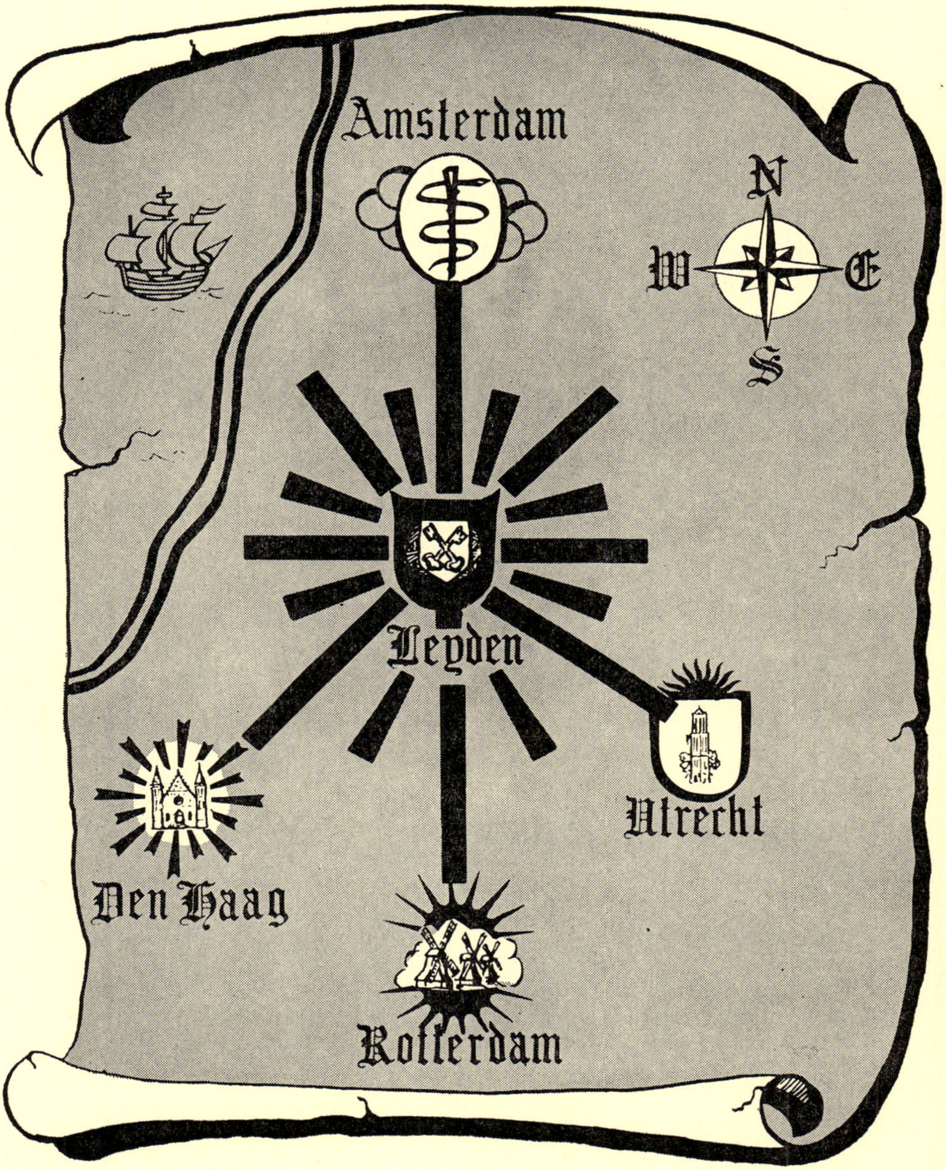


FIGURE 23.

and his illustrious pupils, von Haller and van Swieten, were largely responsible for the teaching which made Leyden so famous.

Herman Boerhaave (1660–1738) was the son of a clergyman. He studied theology at Leyden and had courses in philosophy, mathematics and medicine. After receiving the degree of doctor of philosophy at Leyden, he later decided to become a physician and obtained his doctor of medicine in 1693. His first appointment was as Professor of Medicine. He developed an extensive botanical garden which was

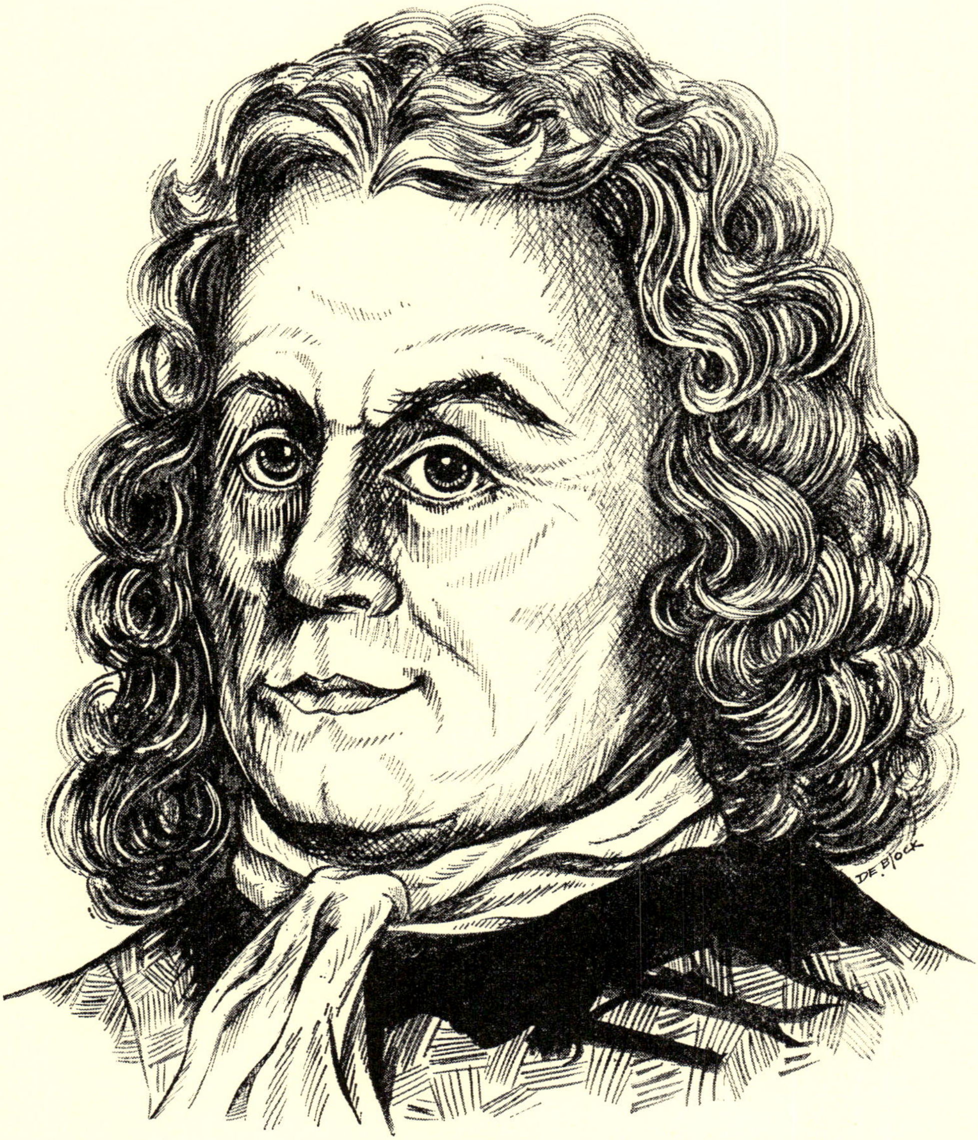


FIGURE 24. Herman Boerhaave of Leyden.

among the first to be in association with a medical institution. His influence is lasting, in spite of the fact that he made no great discoveries in medicine and his writings are forgotten. His influence was based upon his methods of instruction which became a model for institutions in Europe and the foundation for modern clinical teaching. These methods were continued by his illustrious pupils. He had charge of twelve beds for the care of his patients and the teaching of his students and the medical historian, Sigerist, has stated that "on twelve beds half the physicians of Europe were trained." Students from all over Europe flocked to him. He never let his theo-

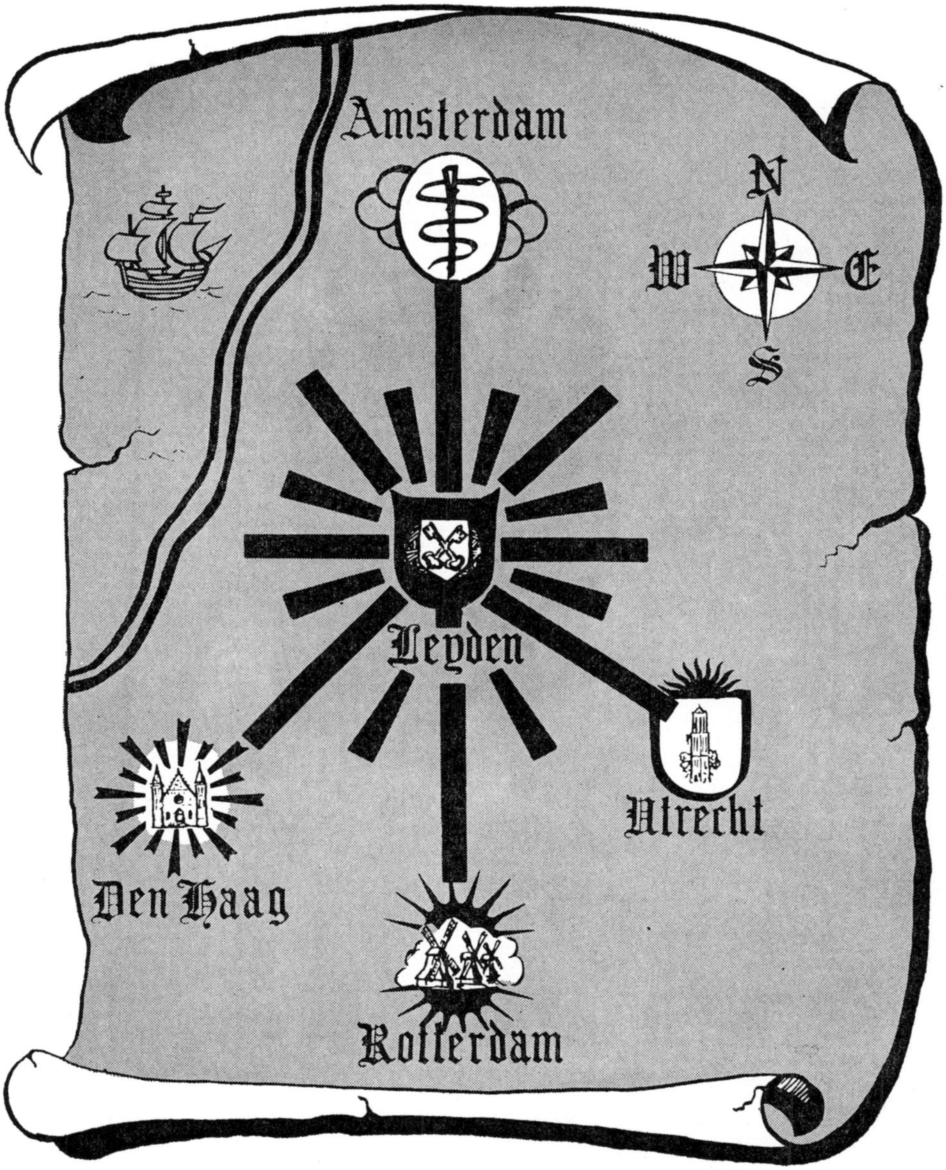


Figure 23.

and his illustrious pupils, von Haller and van Swieten, were largely responsible for the teaching which made Leyden so famous.

Herman Boerhaave (1660–1738) was the son of a clergyman. He studied theology at Leyden and had courses in philosophy, mathematics and medicine. After receiving the degree of doctor of philosophy at Leyden, he later decided to become a physician and obtained his doctor of medicine in 1693. His first appointment was as Professor of Medicine. He developed an extensive botanical garden which was

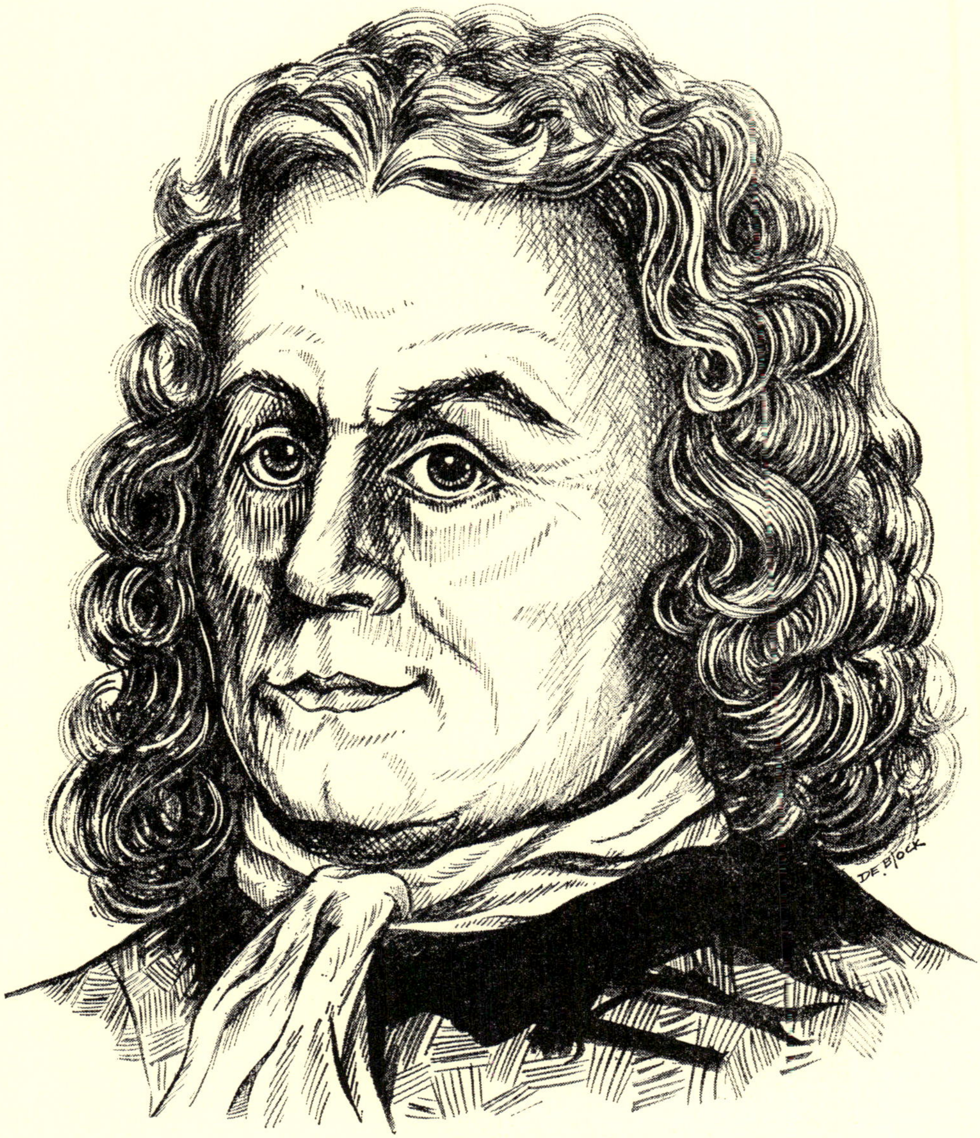

FIGURE 24. Herman Boerhaave of Leyden.

among the first to be in association with a medical institution. His influence is lasting, in spite of the fact that he made no great discoveries in medicine and his writings are forgotten. His influence was based upon his methods of instruction which became a model for institutions in Europe and the foundation for modern clinical teaching. These methods were continued by his illustrious pupils. He had charge of twelve beds for the care of his patients and the teaching of his students and the medical historian, Sigerist, has stated that "on twelve beds half the physicians of Europe were trained." Students from all over Europe flocked to him. He never let his theories conflict with his treatment of patients and placed Sydenham on almost the same plane as Hippocrates.

Albrecht von Haller (1708–1777) was probably the most eminent of the pupils of Boerhaave. He has been referred to as "the greatest systematist after Galen and one of the most imposing figures in all medical history" by Garrison. He was similar to Galen in some respects but he based his medicine upon the foundations of anatomy, physiological observations and experiments. He wrote Latin verses at the age of nine, composed a Greek and Hebrew dictionary as a child and began medicine at the age of fifteen. He also studied in London, Paris and Basel. Boerhaave was his idol. He began practice in Berne, spent seventeen years as Professor of Anatomy, Botany, and Medicine at Göttingen, became homesick and spent the remainder of his life in Berne as the public health officer. Also, von Haller made noteworthy studies in anatomy and embryology. His twelve physiological works included many discoveries which were later forgotten and rediscovered, viz., the myogenic theory of the heartbeat and the role of bile in the digestion of fat. His greatest contribution to physiology was his principle that irritability is a specific property of all muscular tissues and that sensibility is an exclusive property of nervous tissues. As a botanist, he probably has been surpassed only by Linné. His correspondence in the history of science was immense.

Gerhard van Swieten (1700–1772) was possibly the ablest of Boerhaave's assistants and was his logical successor. He was, however, a Roman Catholic and this seemed to be an insurmountable barrier to his progress in Protestant Leyden. Van Swieten accepted the post as physician to the Empress of Vienna and was responsible for the establishment of the Old Vienna School of Medicine.

## THE OLD VIENNA SCHOOL OF MEDICINE

Gerhard van Swieten began to lecture in the court library after accepting the post as physician to the Empress of Vienna. At that time he did not have a university appointment, but Empress Marie Theresa appointed him President of the Medical Faculty of the University in 1748 and charged him with the reformation of the School of Medicine. Prior to this time, although Vienna was the oldest German university except for Prague, its medicine had not developed because of the mediocrity of its faculty. Van Swieten reorganized the School of Medicine and it became state controlled. Appointments were provided by the Empress upon nomination by van Swieten. He met with bitter opposition from the existing faculty but proceeded to establish a botanical garden, a chemical laboratory, a new institute of anatomy and he separated anatomy and surgery. He followed the Leyden tradition. The outstanding physician of the Old Vienna School of Medicine was Auenbrugger who made one of the outstanding contributions to medicine of the eighteenth century.

Leopold Auenbrugger (1722–1809) received his training in Vienna from van Swieten, among others. Auenbrugger was highly successful in medical practice in Vienna, was a lover of music and wrote the libretto for the comic opera *The Chimney Sweep.* His *Inventum Novum* was published in 1761. Although it contained only ninety-five pages, it is considered to be one of the most influential contributions in the history of medicine. Auenbrugger described a new method of physical diagnosis known as percussion. It was based on clinical trial over a period of seven years. It may have been stimulated by his boyhood experiences of learning to estimate the amount of wine in casks by tapping on the ends of wine casks in his father's inn. He described the technique of percussion as well as physical findings in health and disease. His teachers and contemporaries ignored this discovery for the most part. It was popularized forty-seven years later by Jean Corvisart, a famous French physician, who found a reference to Auenbrugger's discovery and published a French translation of *Inventum Novum.* This made Auenbrugger famous. He died the following year.

In the same year (1761) in which Auenbrugger produced *Inventum Novum,* Morgagni of Padua completed work which was to prove itself to be another outstanding contribution to the medicine of the eighteenth century and to the development of pathology.

## THE DEVELOPMENT OF A MODERN CONCEPT OF PATHOLOGY

Giovanni Battista Morgagni (1682–1771) (Fig. 25) published the work that inscribed his name among the greatest in medicine and justly entitled him to be called "The Father of Pathology." His book, *De Sedibus et causis morborum per anatomen indagatis* [*The Seats and Causes of Diseases*], marks the foundation of modern pathological anatomy and one of the influential contributions to medical history. This work introduced anatomical thinking into pathology and localized pathological lesions in definite organs. The author described almost every pathological lesion with which we are familiar today. Morgagni was graduated in medicine from Bologna and became Professor of Medicine at Padua. He became Professor of Anatomy in 1715 and followed the line of Vesalius, Colombo, Fabrizi and other illustrious anatomists. He published texts in 1706, 1717 and 1719 and established his reputation as an anatomist, scholar and master of Latin prose. His masterpiece, *De sedibus,* was published in 1761 when he was seventy-nine years of age and included, for the first time, a vast array of pathological findings all of which were well arranged and indexed. Each description was preceded by a minute history of the disease, the symptoms, the treatment and the relationship between the clinical picture and the autopsy. He described an enormous number of pathological conditions and introduced an anatomical concept into medicine.

Morgagni wrote in the preface:

> So that if any physician observe a singular, or any other symptom in a patient, and desired to know what internal injury is wont to correspond to that symptom; or if an anatomist finds any particular morbid appearance in the dissection of the body, and should wish to know what symptom has preceded an injury of this kind in other bodies; the physician by inspecting the first of these indexes, the anatomist by inspecting the second, will immediately find the observation which contains both (if both have been observed by us).

Morgagni's contribution can be regarded as the culmination of a gradual evolution of pathological anatomy as well as the beginning of the new concept of pathology as it developed in the nineteenth and twentieth centuries.

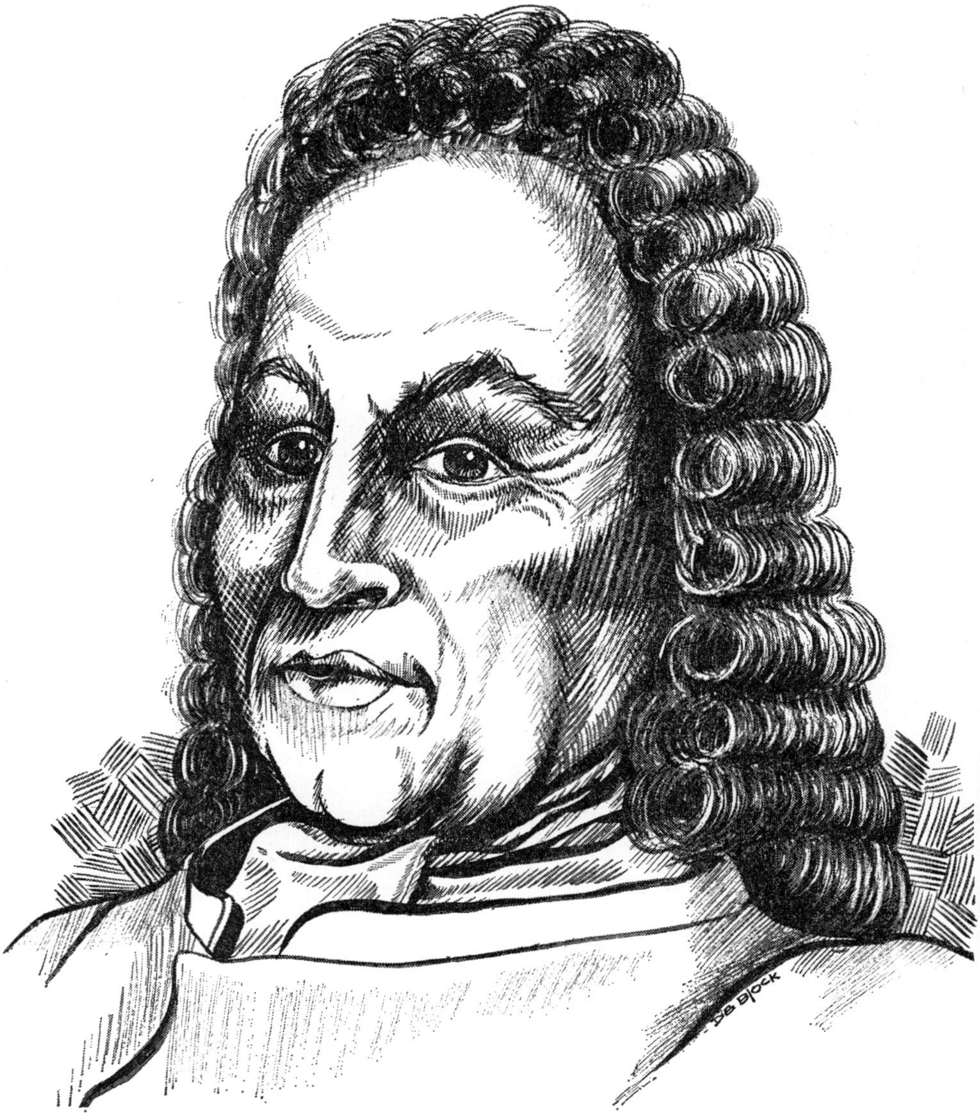

FIGURE 25. Giovanni Battista Morgagni—"Father of Pathology."

Galen had said: "There are very few essential symptoms of disease which do not point to the affected part. Indeed the alterations of functions indicate only the affected area." In turn Galen's advocacy of anatomy had its roots in the Alexandrian School of Medicine where, five hundred years before him, anatomy of the human body was freely practiced and taught by Herophilus and Erasistratus. These pioneers in turn, might have been inspired by Hippocrates.

In his book on ancient medicine, Hippocrates stated:

I am further convinced that it is necessary to know what sufferings come to a man from powers and what from shapes. I mean, roughly, by power an extreme sense of humor by shapes the various forms to be found among the parts of the body.

Berengario da Carpi, in his commentaries in 1521 on Mondino's *Anatomy*, invokes the authority of Averroes who maintained that

> Internal diseases require signs to manifest themselves and their causes. They are recognized by impaired function and impairment of function is perceived by knowledge of the normal operation of the parts of the body and such knowledge can only be acquired by competent anatomy.

Boerhaave wrote in 1728 that

> In spite of most detailed description of all disease phenomena, one does not know anything of the cause until one has opened the body.

The organization of hospitals and autopsies was an important factor contributory to the advancement of clinical anatomic investigation. The ultimate development derived from Morgagni's fundamental principle and Auenbrugger's vision came nearly a hundred years later with visualization of organ alteration by roentgen rays. It was Morgagni's aim to provide medicine with a complete lexicon defining clinical symptoms in terms of organ lesions. This endeavor promoted greater accuracy, anatomic investigation, and accentuated the importance of more penetrating observations at the bedside. It is no coincidence that physiological research rose in importance and scope for scientific medicine.

Johannes Müller wrote in 1836 the following words

> May the genius already be born who will create for us a general pathology founded upon physiology and pathological anatomy, worthy of the state of our sciences of medicine and of nature.

This prophecy became true some twenty years later with the publication of Virchow's *Cellularpathologie*. Virchow shared with Morgagni the belief that disease was localized, yet not within organs only but within the cells of the body. His pathogenic concept differed from that of Morgagni because of the advances of science and technology.

Meanwhile a new medical school of the first rank developed at the University of Edinburgh from earlier beginnings.

## THE UNIVERSITY OF EDINBURGH

The faculty of Town's College, and Doctor Archibald Pitcairne (1652–1713), established the School of Medicine at the University of Edinburgh in 1685. Doctor Pitcairne was called to Leyden in 1692 as Professor of Medicine, taught Boerhaave and later returned to Edinburgh.

For 126 years (1720–1846) the professorship of anatomy in the medical school at Edinburgh was held by an Alexander Monro—three generations of the same family—and they were associated with much of the early fame of the medical school.

*Alexander Monro* was appointed Professor of Anatomy in the Medical School of the University of Edinburgh in 1720 when he was twenty-two years of age. He was a skilled anatomist and an excellent teacher. His father had been an army surgeon who had been trained at Leyden by Pitcairne, and he himself was a pupil of his father's contemporary, Boerhaave and had also been trained at Leyden.

He was succeeded by his son, Alexander Monro, in 1758 who actually surpassed him as a teacher and as an anatomist. Among his many contributions, he described the openings between the lateral ventricles of the brain into the third ventricle. These are known today as the foramina of Monro. He carried out many anatomical investigations on the lymphatics and on the nervous system.

The third Alexander Monro succeeded his father in 1808, was less successful than his predecessors and taught until 1846.

William Cullen (1710–1790) contributed greatly to raise Edinburgh to the rank of first medical school in Europe, a position which it long held. He attracted students to Edinburgh from England and the colonies as Boerhaave had drawn them to Leyden. Cullen rivaled Sydenham for his descriptions and classifications of diseases but made no very original contributions. His pupil and secretary was John Brown.

John Brown (1735–1788) taught that phenomena of life depended upon excitability and that disease results from a local or generalized increase or decrease of excitability. On this basis, he divided patients into two groups: those who were sthenic and had increased excitability and therefore required sedatives for treatment, and those who were asthenic and had decreased excitability and therefore required stimulants for treatment. Brown's favorite remedies were whiskey and laudanum and he became addicted to both. His followers were known as Brunonians. They were noisy, argumentative and actually had warfare with the Cullenites on occasion. He made few converts in Great Britain and created little interest in France but became strong in Germany. Benjamin Rush of Philadelphia was impressed by Brown. Two other physicians from Edinburgh of this period were Pringle and Lind.

Sir John Pringle was born in 1707, was trained by Boerhaave in Leyden and then settled in Edinburgh. He was sent to Flanders with the British Army and placed in charge of a military hospital. After returning to London, he became a member of the Royal Society and physician to the King. His work earned him the title of "The Founder of Modern Military Medicine." His treatise was called *Observations on the Diseases of the Army*. It was published in 1752 and laid down basic principles of military sanitation and stressed proper ventilation.

James Lind (1716–1794) wrote three classics on scurvy, naval hygiene and tropical diseases in 1753, 1757, and 1768, respectively. He recommended the use of lemon juice in the prevention and cure of scurvy. Unfortunately, he died without seeing any of his suggestions officially adopted by the British Navy. In 1794, the year of his death, lemon juice was used on a long cruise and prevented scurvy entirely. The use of lemons and lemon juice became standard in the rations of sailors later and, as a result, scurvy disappeared from the British Navy. British sailors are still known as "Limeys" because of this treatment. Lind had been with the navy for nine years prior to obtaining his doctor of medicine degree at the University of Edinburgh. He practiced there and then in naval hospitals. The British Navy estimated that, in a period of twenty years prior to Lind and his discovery, it had lost ten thousand mariners with scurvy which became known as the "calamity of sailors."

A number of outstanding physicians and surgeons provided major contributions to the medicine of the eighteenth century in England and wrote in the true spirit of Hippocrates after studying their patients at the bedside. Some of these individuals were Heberden, Baker, the Hunters, Withering and Jenner.

## SOME ENGLISH CLINICIANS OF THE EIGHTEENTH CENTURY

William Heberden (1710–1801) provided the first clear description of angina pectoris, a description of Heberden's nodes and one of the earliest accounts of chickenpox in English. His work was published in his *Commentaries on the History and Cure of Diseases* in 1802 both in Latin and in English.

Sir George Baker (1722–1809) like Heberden, was another scholar from Cambridge University. Baker observed that colic was common in Devon and rare in Hereford. He noted that farmers in Devon used lead-lined cider presses and that lead could be extracted from this cider but not from that made in Hereford. After removing the lead lining from the cider presses, his fellow Devonshire townsmen no longer had colic. He read his famous *Inquiry Concerning the Causes of the Endemic Colic of Devonshire* before the Royal College of Physicians in 1767.

Caleb Parry (1755–1822) gave the first clear account of exophthalmic goiter. He described eight patients in all, the first one being observed in 1786. He was a graduate of Edinburgh and wrote one of the earliest accounts of angina pectoris which he attributed to disease of the coronary arteries. His account of goiter appeared in his *Unpublished Medical Writings* in 1825.

William Hunter (1718–1783) labored for a period of thirty years in order to publish his greatest scientific achievement, *The Anatomy of the Gravid Uterus,* in 1774. This text contained thirty-four, life-sized, anatomically exact and artistically perfect plates. William Hunter was born in Scotland, studied for the ministry during a period of five years in Glasgow, apprenticed for three years to William Cullen, attended lectures by Monro and then went to London. At first he lived with Doctor Smellie who was a countryman and just beginning his career as an obstetrician. Young Hunter became an anatomist, lectured on anatomy and began his practice as an obstetrician in 1748. He delivered Queen Charlotte's son who became King George IV. His home included a lecture theater, dissecting rooms, museum and a remarkable collection of specimens. He demonstrated the lacrimal ducts in 1747 and the seminiferous tubules with the assistance of his younger brother John in 1752.

John Hunter (1728–1793) was ten years younger than William. John (Fig. 26) was spoiled by an indulgent mother and received an imperfect education but did show considerable skill in dissection after he went to London to work in his brother's dissection rooms. He demonstrated the branches of the olfactory nerves and also the previously unknown branches of the fifth nerve. He was able to show the course of the arteries of the gravid uterus and the presence of lymphatic vessels in birds. He ultimately felt he received inadequate credit from his brother and they became estranged. John Hunter joined the army in 1760 and had considerable experience with gunshot wounds. He began his practice as a surgeon in 1763 and continued to lecture on anatomy and surgery in London. Because he was not articulate and his basic education was incomplete, he fortified himself on laudanum. In spite of this he became a great teacher and attracted a

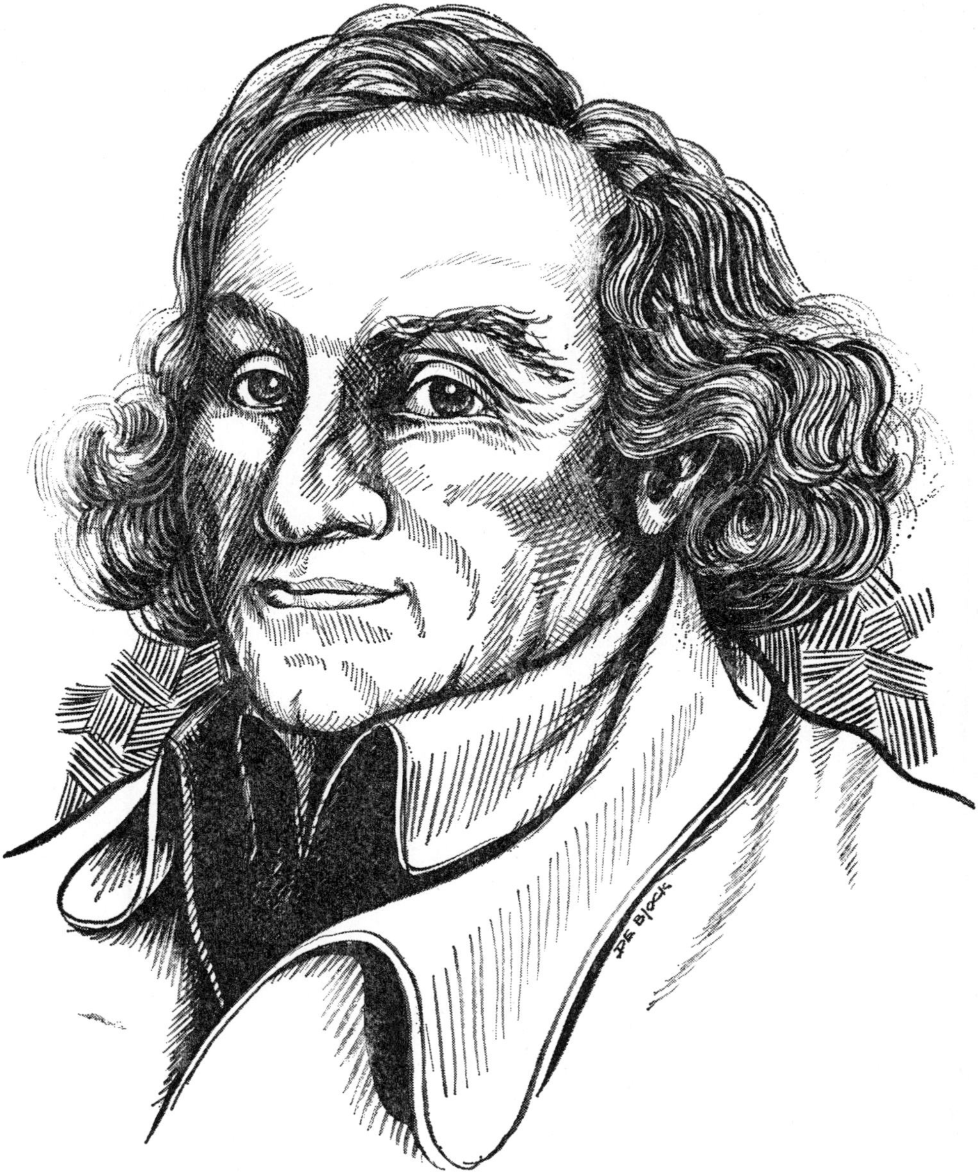


FIGURE 26. John Hunter—pioneer of physiological surgery.

group of brilliant pupils who later became famous (Brillie, Cooper, Abernathy, Howe, Physick and Jenner). His surgical progress was slow and his chief interest was his museum of natural history. However, his reputation as an anatomist, naturalist and investigator spread rapidly. He became surgeon to St. George's Hospital in 1769, Surgeon-Extraordinary to the King in 1776 and Surgeon-General of the Army in 1789.

John Hunter published four classics: (1) *The Natural History of the Human Teeth,* in 1771. This was the first scientific treatise on dentistry in the English language and included anatomy, physiology, diseases, and the principle that a tooth can be moved slowly by pressure (orthodonture), (2) *A Treatise on Venereal Disease,* in 1786. In 1767, Hunter had inoculated himself with pus from a patient with gonorrhea in order to determine whether the poison of gonorrhea was identical with that of syphilis. He developed gonorrhea and a chancre. He described the latter and this subsequently was called a "hunterian chancre." He treated himself with mercury for three years and considered himself cured. He obviously had both diseases and made the error that gonorrhea and syphilis were the same, (3) *Observations on Certain Parts of the Animal Economy,* in 1786 and (4) *Treatise on Blood Inflammation and Gunshot Wounds* in 1794.

Hunter carried out many experiments in an attempt to solve the problems that he encountered in his practice. He had an attack of epigastric angina in 1773 and for the next twenty years had periodic angina pectoris. Hunter remarked that his life was in the hands of any rascal who chose to annoy or to tease him. After a dispute at a board meeting at St. George's Hospital, he died during an attack of angina pectoris. Surgery was truly an operative science at the time that John Hunter entered this field. It is to his credit that he made it a physiological science as well.

Two additional contributions of significance were made in the second half of the eighteenth century: Withering and Jenner provided new and decisive principles of medical treatment.

William Withering (1741–1799) introduced digitalis which still remains as a basic medication in the management of heart disease. He was a graduate of Edinburgh, practiced medicine in Birmingham and was an ardent student of botany. His first work was *A Botanical Arrangement of all the Vegetables Naturally Growing in Great Britain* (1766). His classic, *An Account of the Foxglove and Some of its Medicinal Uses,* appeared with a beautiful color plate of digitalis purpurae in 1785. Withering had heard of an old woman in Shropshire who had a secret remedy for the cure of dropsy. He was able to obtain the recipe and analysis showed it to contain twenty or more herbs, the active one being foxglove. He used foxglove therapy for a period of ten years before his publication. The active ingredient of foxglove is digitalis.

Edward Jenner (1749–1823) discovered vaccination for smallpox. He was educated in the classics and was later apprenticed to a physician near Bristol for a period of six years. During his apprenticeship he was called in consultation to see a young woman who was responsible for giving him the clue to the importance of vaccination. When smallpox was mentioned, she exclaimed: "I cannot take it, for I have had cowpox." He went on to London in order to become a pupil of John Hunter and lived in his home for two years. He became one of Hunter's favorite pupils but also tired of London and spent the remainder of his life in rural practice and in experimentation in Berkeley. He made observations on hedgehogs, lizards, birds, and foxes and on the cuckoo. Because of this work he was elected a Fellow of the Royal Society of London.

Smallpox was considered to be one of the major scourges of the human race before Jenner made it possible for it to be prevented. He obtained some pus from a sore on a dairymaid's hand and inserted it by means of a superficial incision in the arm of a healthy eight-year-old boy (James Phipps). The inoculation succeeded and the boy developed a small pustular sore, scab and scar. Jenner inoculated him with variola (smallpox) lymph six weeks later and smallpox did not occur. He inoculated three more patients during the next year (1797) and submitted a paper on the subject to the council of the Royal Society. The manuscript was returned to him with the "friendly admonition that as he had gained some reputation by his former papers it was not advisable to present this one." He went ahead and published it himself in 1798 under the title *The Inquiry into the Causes and Effects of the Variolae Vaccinae.*

Jenner's discovery and London publication created much controversy. It was accepted abroad before it was accepted at home. The work was enthusiastically supported in America by Doctor Benjamin Waterhouse who was Professor of Theory and Practice of Medicine at the Medical School of Harvard College.* President Thomas Jefferson, Napoleon and the Empress of Russia also supported vaccination and the method spread generally thereafter. Disfigurement and death from small pox were commonplace in the eighteenth century. Finally, in countries which enforced compulsory vaccination, the death rate approached zero. The discovery of vaccination by Jenner ranks among the greatest advances in medical history.

Some outstanding discoveries in physiology and chemistry were also made during this period.

* The work of Doctor Waterhouse is discussed in Chapter XVII.

## ADVANCES IN PHYSIOLOGY AND CHEMISTRY DURING THE EIGHTEENTH CENTURY

In keeping with major scientific discovery of any period, the work of many predecessors and unusual preparation and industry on the part of the current investigators made advances possible in physiology and chemistry during the eighteenth century.

### Physiology

The outstanding English physiologist during the eighteenth century was the Rev. Stephen Hales (1677–1761). He was educated at Cambridge University as a divinity student and became interested in biology, chemistry, physical science, astronomy and did some dissections in anatomy and experiments in physiology. He settled in Teddington, a village with a population of approximately five hundred people which was located fifteen miles from London. He became the "perpetual curate" to the people of Teddington and also began to experiment in his free time. He was very active in all respects until his death at the age of eighty-four.

His classic experiment was to record an estimation of blood pressure for the first time. This was done in 1711. He placed a brass tube in the crural artery of a horse and attached an upright glass tube which was nine feet in length. He then untied the ligature on the artery and observed blood to rise in the tube for a distance of eight feet and three inches above the level of the left ventricle of the heart. This experiment as well as others led to his election as Fellow of the Royal Society in 1718.

The physiology of digestion and respiration also benefited by significant discoveries during the eighteenth century, particularly by the work of de Reaumur and Spallanzani.

René de Réaumur (1683–1767) prepared an important landmark in the history of digestion in 1752. He was a lawyer by training and devoted himself to scientific investigations in Paris and was elected to the Academy of Sciences in 1708. His treatise on the digestion of birds gave great impetus to subsequent studies of digestion. His experimental animal was the kite because this bird rejects from its stomach things that it has swallowed but cannot digest. He fed meals, introduced sponges which were rejected, and studied the gastric juices. He was able to discover the power of digestion of gastric juice and that digestion was not just a matter of trituration and putrefaction as had been assumed. He demonstrated that gastric juice actually had the power to dissolve food.

Lazzaro Spallanzani (1729–1799) extended the studies of Réamur. He showed that all tissues respire. He demolished the doctrine of spontaneous generation by demonstrating under the microscope that no signs of life developed in water that was boiled and sealed in a flask unless the seal had been broken and air was permitted to enter. This work was done in 1767.

## Chemistry

Developments in chemistry during the eighteenth century included those provided by Black, Cavendish, Priestley, Scheele and Lavoisier and led to the discovery of oxygen.

Joseph Black (1728–1799) was the founder of *calorimetry*, the measurement of heat, and he introduced the doctrine of latent heat. He showed that when lime is burned it becomes caustic or quicklime, and loses weight, and that this weight loss is due to the loss of a specific gas. He believed this gas was the same as that given off in fermentation, burning charcoal and in expired air. His work contradicted the prevailing phlogiston theory that lime becomes caustic by taking out the substance called phlogiston and should be heavier in this state.

Henry Cavendish (1731–1810) prepared hydrogen by treating iron with acids in 1766, and water by burning hydrogen with oxygen * in 1781. He showed that atmospheric air contains a mixture of oxygen and nitrogen in constant proportions. Cavendish further undermined the phlogiston theory and yet tried to harmonize his results with it.

Joseph Priestley (1733–1804) described his tests with "fixed air, inflammable air, and nitrous air which he discovered." Carbon dioxide, hydrogen, and nitrous oxide are the terms presently applied to these three gases. Priestley discovered hydrochloric acid gas and obtained "dephlogisticated air" by heating mercuric oxide with a burning glass. This gas was not flammable but did support combustion. His interpretation was that air supported combustion because it takes up the phlogiston given off by the burning body. He actually discovered oxygen without understanding it and championed the phlogiston theory in spite of the mounting evidence against it. His experiments, however, were excellent.

Karl Scheele (1742–1786) obtained "fire air" by heating red oxide of mercury, and from black oxide of mercury and saltpeter in 1772. He was another devoted fol-

* Oxygen was discovered in 1777 by Lavoisier.

lower of the phlogiston theory but in reality destroyed it without recognizing the real importance of his discoveries.

Antoine Lavoisier (1743–1794) will be remembered as the "Father of Modern Chemistry," the destroyer of the phlogiston theory and for discoveries in the field of respiration comparable to those of Harvey in circulation. He was a brilliant and well-educated Parisian. His thesis on street-lighting was completed when he was twenty-four and he was elected to the Academy of Sciences. He established his own laboratory in which he worked full-time on experimentation, particularly in chemistry. His publication, *On the Nature of the Principle which Combines with Metals During Calcination,* appeared in 1775. In it, he described how a metal, when burned into oxide, increased in weight by taking something from the air. Lavoisier conclusively showed in 1777 that substances which had been called "dephlogisticated air" combined with metals when calcined and that this property was characteristic of acids. He proposed the name *oxygen* (generator of acid) for such substances. He gave Priestley full credit for making the material first. Historians and Priestley have given Lavoisier the full credit for proving the fallacy of the phlogiston theory and understanding the true meaning of oxygen.

Lavoisier recognized that respiration was oxidation in which oxygen disappears on inspiration and carbon dioxide appears on expiration. He published on respiration in 1777 and in 1790. His last contribution in 1790 was suppressed because of the French Revolution. Antoine Lavoisier was charged with being an enemy of France for "mixing tobacco with water and ingredients harmful to the health of the citizens" and was executed by the guillotine on the following day (May 9, 1794).

The eighteenth century closed with interest in electricity and a new system known as "mesmerism."

## ELECTRICITY AND MESMERISM

*Electricity* is a term derived from the Greek word for amber. Thales as early as 600 B.C. had observed that one could attract light objects to yellow amber if it had been rubbed first. Many experiments with electricity occurred during the sixteenth, seventeenth and eighteenth centuries and medical electricity was discussed by Joseph Priestley in his text, *History and Present State of Electricity*. Benjamin Franklin treated paralysis with electrical currents, De Haen used electric shocks to treat St. Vitus dance and Rev. John Wesley made use of electricity in treating patients.

Franz Anton Mesmer (1734–1815) proposed his doctrine of disease in his doctoral thesis, *On the Influence of Planets.* His concept was that planets attract each other and also exercise a direct influence on the human body by means of a mysterious fluid termed "animal magnetism." His claims were investigated by a committee from the Academy of Sciences including Benjamin Franklin and Antoine Lavoisier. Their conclusions were that animal magnetic fluid was nonexistent, and that the effects claimed by Mesmer were produced entirely by the imagination of his patients. Puységur was one of Mesmer's disciples and developed a technique for producing hypnosis in 1784. Although hypnotism has been known in one form or another since early times, mesmerism and hypnotism became almost synonymous and the practice spread widely. Although Mesmer has remained a spiritual ancestor for later cults which utilize seances and other similar practices, hypnotism has become established in psychiatric medicine.

## SUMMARY

The eighteenth century provided an imposing group of clinicians. These individuals made careful observations of disease and studied various methods of treatment in an age that was very conscious of its intellectual emancipation and intent upon applying new ideas in practice. Physical diagnosis was placed on a firm basis by the discovery of percussion. Pathology was founded as a modern science. Physiology and chemistry developed and witnessed the discovery of oxygen. Vaccination was introduced and made possible the prevention of one of the worst scourges of the human race.

*Man can do a great deal by observation and thinking, but with them alone he cannot unravel the mysteries of nature.*—Sir William Osler

# XVI European Medicine of the First Half of the Nineteenth Century

During the first half of the nineteenth century,* Paris was the unquestioned leader of medicine in the world. Europe was involved in a struggle between liberal and republican movements against monarchies and remnants of feudalism. Peoples who had long been under alien domination developed strong nationalist feelings. The early years of the nineteenth century saw Napoleon Bonaparte as the leading figure, and the format and aftereffects of the French Revolution actually dominated the Continent of Europe during the first half of the nineteenth century. The growth of urbanization and industrialization of the countries of Europe also changed the social structure of these nations. New empires developed with the expansion of English, French and Russian possessions.

Inventions of the eighteenth and nineteenth centuries made possible an unprecedented development of iron and textile industries and started an industrial revolution. Industrialization which began in England and gradually spread to Germany, America and then to the rest of Europe, converted a rural peasantry into an urban industrial society. Such inventions as the steam engine in 1769, methods for using coal in blast furnaces, railways, machines for making textiles, the rise of engineering and the discovery and utilization of electricity contributed to this change. The reaction to the Industrial Revolution took many forms from the smashing of machinery to the development of modern socialism.

Urbanization, with its overcrowding, unsanitary housing conditions, and lack of proper supervision of the water and food supply made life in these newly industrialized and congested centers hazardous from the standpoint of health. These problems were the seeds for the concept that public health is a responsibility of the State as well as the individual. The term "Father of Public Health" has been bestowed on Johann Peter Frank (1745–1821). His text, *Medicine Administered by the State,* began to appear in 1779, with the third volume being published in 1783 and a fourth in 1795. These were the first com-

* The history of the nineteenth century is so lacking in homogeneity that it is more easily understood if considered under three consecutive headings: (1) European medicine of the first half of the nineteenth century, (2) American medicine before the second half of the nineteenth century, and (3) Medicine during the second half of the nineteenth century.

prehensive treatises on public health and discussed in detail such subjects as vital statistics, marital hygiene, infant and maternal mortality, child welfare, infectious diseases, food inspection and sanitation. His work was excellent, but, like the Austrian thinking of the period, was fixed and absolute. He became the director of the Allgemeines Krankenhaus and Professor of Medicine in the University of Vienna in 1795. His medical clinic was outstanding in Europe. Beethoven, the son of Napoleon, and the Czar of Russia were among his patients. During his lifetime he was famed as a skilled physician and teacher and only later did his public health recommendations take root and spread.

Humanitarianism and reformers emerged in every field of life during this period. Slavery was abolished in the British Empire in 1833, a Factory Act made it illegal for children to work more than ten hours a day and societies were developed for the prevention of cruelty to children. Many missionary societies were established in order to improve the lives and morals of people in the Orient, Africa and elsewhere because of their acceptance of the principle that all men are brothers.

Romanticism was characteristic of the literature of the first half of the nineteenth century with the poetry of Byron, Shelley, Heine and the romances of Dumas and Scott. A broad spectrum of philosophies was propounded during this period. The cult of individualism based on the doctrine that the ego is the source of all experience (Fichte) was popular and von Schelling saw history as a series of stages progressing toward a general harmony. Hegel regarded history as a result of an interplay of forces leading to a synthesis. Thus, the schools of social and political thought varied from that of the organized state being the expression of the highest human idealism and the finest good of mankind, to those who felt that all forms of government and property ownership were evil and should be abolished.

The early years of the nineteenth century witnessed a constant succession of brilliant physicians and great surgeons in France. In this regard the medical historian Major has commented:

> It seemed as if the God of Medicine which had once had his habitation in Greece, then wandered to Alexandria, from there to Baghdad, then to Italy during the Renaissance, to the Netherlands, had now taken up his abode in Paris.

## THE PARIS SCHOOL OF MEDICINE

Other factors than Napoleon * himself probably should be taken into consideration for the ascendency of French medicine. It is more likely that the new France, because of its political liberty and individual rights, had created a state favorable for economic expansion and orderly government and made it possible for outstanding individuals in the arts and sciences to develop. Some of the great figures in the history of medicine belong to what has been called the Paris School, including Bichat, Magendie, Cruveilhier, Broussais, Laennec, Corvisart, Bouilland, Boyle, Louis, Larry and Dupuytren.

Marie-Francois Bichat (1771–1802) has been described as the "Father of Descrip-

* In reality, disease did much to defeat Napoleon's army. He started with 400,000 men in his Russian campaign and returned with only 3,000 having lost the majority from diseases such as typhus and typhoid fevers. These diseases were spread upon the return of the surviving soldiers to central Europe.

tive Anatomy." His work was possibly the most fruitful legacy to the budding nineteenth century because of his idea that the living body was not merely made up of organs but could be studied on the basis of an intricate network of tissues ("membranes"). He began his professional career as a surgeon and then turned to anatomy and physiology. He performed more than six hundred autopsies during one winter. He died prematurely at the age of thirty-one, presumably of overwork. His work, *General Anatomy,* was published in 1801 and contained detailed descriptions of the body in health and disease. Pathologists had previously emphasized the organs of the body and Bichat stressed the importance of the systems, such as the cellular tissues, the arteries, the veins, lymphatics, bones, muscles and glands in the diseased state. This work had great influence on medicine and is reflected in the writings of Broussais, Corvisart, Laennec and led directly to the cellular theory of Virchow some decades later.

Francois Magendie (1783–1855) was unquestionably the initiator of the movement to devote full time to experimental medicine. Other physicians in the past, notably Galen and Harvey, had experimented, but none so systematically nor to the exclusion of clinical practice. Thus, in the first half of the century, physiology finally freed itself from metaphysical speculation and became a science based upon experimental research. Magendie's first paper in 1809 laid down "distrust of theory and firm faith in experiment." When he described the effects of poison on animals before the Paris Academie de Sciences in 1809, the beginning of experimental pharmacology was made. He founded the first periodical which was devoted exclusively to physiology. He made the first observation of anaphylaxis in 1839, when he observed that rabbits might tolerate a single injection of egg albumin but often died following the second injection. His greatest contribution was probably that the anterior spinal nerves are motor, and the posterior spinal nerves are sensory, in function. This was established on the basis of experimentation in 1822. Sir Charles Bell had carried out experiments thirteen years earlier, unknown to Magendie, and had noted convulsive movements produced by anterior root stimulation. Bell regarded himself primarily as an anatomist and had a distaste for experimental work. The question of priority has been revived again and again. Physiologists generally give Magendie the most credit. The designation "Bell-Magendie Rule" is now accepted in medical literature to indicate the direction of conduction in the spinal nerve roots.

Jean Cruveilhier (1791–1874) was the first to hold the newly established chair of pathology at the University of Paris. He held this position from 1836 for a period of thirty years. He was also physician to the Salpétriere and the Charité. His atlas was published with unsurpassed illustrations, mostly in color and artistically perfect. Cruveilhier made the first description and illustration of disseminated sclerosis, an early description of progressive muscular atrophy, and he pictured several cases of gastric ulcer. Gastric ulcer is still called "la maladie de Cruveilhier" by the French.

Francois Broussais (1772–1838) was a noted clinician and Professor of General Pathology in Paris. He was powerful, dogmatic and a great lecturer. His *Physiological Medicine* did not consider disease

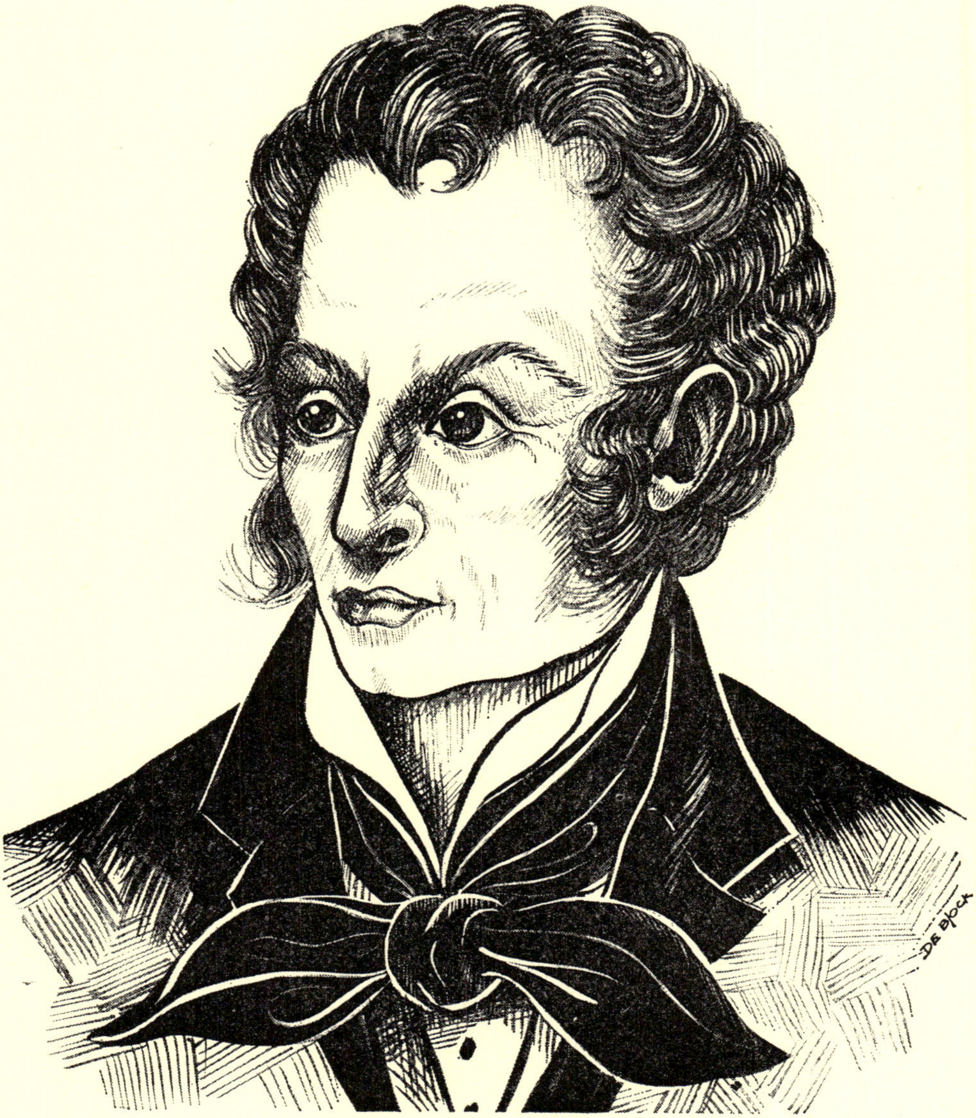


FIGURE 27. René Theophile Laennec—discoverer of the stethoscope.

entities or anatomical changes, but rather irritability of tissues. He held that all disease was a chemical reaction to excessive stimuli and that inflammation was transmitted from the intestine. He believed in therapeutic starvation and used leeches extensively for the purpose of reducing the amount of blood in the body. It has been said that during this period importation of leeches in France increased from two or three million to over forty million per year. He was one of Laénnec's most determined adversaries.

Rene Theophile Laénnec (1781–1826) was an expert pathologist and a skillful physician (Fig. 27). He was appointed as physician to the Necker Hospital in 1814. It was he who invented the stethoscope in

1816 and wrote one of the important publications in medical history in 1819 regarding its use.

The term *stethoscope* is believed to be of Greek derivation meaning "to look at the chest." He obtained the idea of a stethoscope while walking in the courtyard of the Louvre where he observed some children at play. Their play consisted of listening to the transmission of the sound of pins striking one another at one end of long, hollowed pieces of wood. The following morning he rolled a sheet of paper and tied it up with string and then listened to the heart of a patient at the Necker Hospital. He observed the magnification of the sounds of the heart. He was an expert wood-turner so he produced some twelve-inch cylinders which were hollowed and divided in the middle so that the two parts could be separated and carried (Fig. 28). This became the first stethoscope and led to his publication which summed up eighteen years of medical experience as well as three years of work with the instrument. His treatise covered diseases of the lungs and of the heart. Laénnec was obliged to create a number of new words for the sounds he heard. These words are commonplace today and include râles, bronchophony, pectoriloquy, egophony. His work was immediately accepted. The second edition appeared in 1826.* He died of tuberculosis at the age of forty-five. Laénnec was Corvisart's most famous pupil.

Jean Nicholas Corvisart (1755–1821) was the premiere physician of this period. He became Professor of Practical Medicine in the College de France in 1797, and this appointment was considered to be the highest teaching honor in France. He examined patients carefully and employed the new method of percussion of Auenbrugger. His publication on cardiac disease in 1806 became the outstanding book on the subject of its time. In this treatise he classified diseases of the heart according to their anatomic location, i.e., diseases of the pericardium, heart muscle, endocardium and valves. He used the term *organic lesion* and also distinguished between hypertrophy and dilation of the heart and between right and left heart failure. He also described with accuracy mitral and aortic valvular lesions and tricuspid stenosis. He casually referred to the coronary arteries but did not mention angina pectoris. His translation of Auenbrugger's *Inventum Novum* was published in Paris in 1808 and Corvisart added to this his own observations based upon "long experience with percussion." This work rescued Auenbrugger and his contribution on percussion from ill-merited oblivion. In addition to Laennec, Corvisart had a number of other famous pupils including Bayle and Bouillaud.

Gaspard Bayle (1774–1815) published his *Research on Pulmonary Phthisis* in 1810 when he was thirty-six years of age. He pointed out that a tubercle may be present in patients before symptoms appear and was able to correlate tubercles with the formation of cavities. Bayle described miliary tuberculosis, tubercular laryngitis, lymphadenitis and enteritis. He insisted that tuberculosis was a specific disease and not a degenerative condition which followed other diseases. He died of tuberculosis at the age of forty-two.

Pierre Charles Alexander Louis (1787–1872) was educated in Paris and practiced

* The title of this publication was *Traité de l'auscultation médiate.*

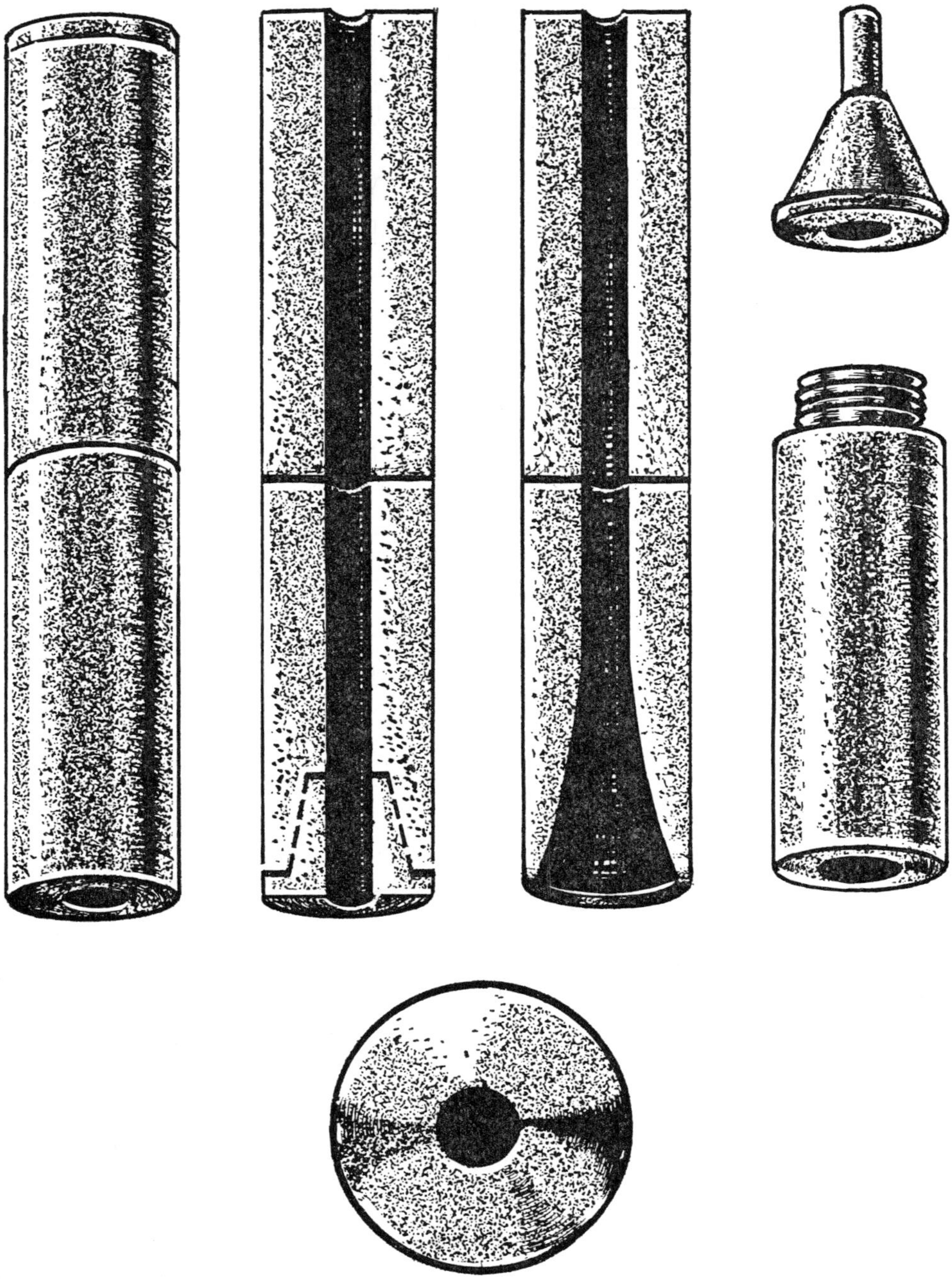

FIGURE 28. Laennec's stethoscope.

in Odessa. Following a severe diphtheria epidemic he resolved to give up practice to study and did so for a period of seven years between the ages of thirty-three and forty. He worked at the Charite in Paris. His observations were published with great care and accuracy on one hundred twenty-three cases of tuberculosis in 1825. He showed specific intestinal lesions in typhoid fever in 1829. His research on the effect of blood-letting, and the demonstration that this procedure never arrested an attack of pneumonia, and that its beneficial effect upon the course of the disease was difficult to prove was published in 1835.

Jean Bouillaud (1790–1881) was a pupil of Corvisart, Laennec, Dupuytren and Magendie. He made significant contributions in the fields of the nervous system and cardiology. His experiments were controlled by clinical and autopsy findings. In a paper published in 1825, he confirmed the view of Gall that the center for articulate speech is located in the anterior lobes of the brain, and pointed out the difference between the ability to create words and the ability to articulate them. He was the first accurately to describe and name the endocardium and endocarditis. He noted the changes in endocarditis beginning with exudation and terminating in cicatricization (scarring) and deformity of the valves. His publications on these subjects in 1835 and in 1836 also elucidated the association between endocarditis and acute articular rheumatism, the mechanism and significance of normal and abnormal heart sounds and rhythms and corrected some of Laennec's errors.

Philippe Pinel (1755–1826) will be remembered by posterity as a great psychiatrist. He had been deeply moved when a friend who was insane ran away into the forest and was devoured by wolves. This led him to study mental diseases. He had attained such ability in this field by 1792 that he was appointed as the physician to the Bicêtre, a hospital for the insane. He found many of the patients in chains, being treated like animals and shown for a price to curiosity seekers. Because of this state of affairs, he introduced humane methods of treatment and published a text in 1801. This publication is a landmark in the history of mental disorders with systematization of twenty-seven hundred mental diseases into classes, orders, genera and species. This was artificial in that it followed the lead of Carl von Linne (1707–1770), the founder of modern botany, and his classification has subsequently been replaced by better work. A statue of Pinel stands today in the park in front of the Salpêtriere.

In the first half of the nineteenth century surgeons used techniques which were not much different from those of Ambroise Paré of the sixteenth century, but they were more thoroughly versed in anatomy and pathology. Speed and daring were considered among the qualifications for brilliance in surgery. Two outstanding surgeons of Paris were Dupuytren and Larrey.

Guillaume Dupuytren (1777–1834) achieved eminence because of long and careful training in anatomy, pathology and surgery. His achievements were numerous. He devised an entertome to be used in making an artificial anus; was the first to successfully remove the lower jaw; sectioned the sternomastoid muscle for wry neck; first successfully ligated the external iliac vessel, and named the condition in the hand now known as Dupuytren's contracture and cured it by operation. His works were published by his pupils in 1830–1834, translated and disseminated widely. He had a violent quarrel with Laennec because the latter resented Dupuytren's attempts to belittle Bichat and to appropriate Bichat's work. His maxim was, "Nothing should be feared so much for a man as mediocrity."

He lived and died true to this and was more respected than loved.

Dominique Larrey (1766–1842) was one of the great surgeons of the early nineteenth century. He was educated in Paris and spent most of his active days as an army surgeon and rose to prominence by sheer force of character and ability. He became a devoted friend of Napoleon and was with him during the campaigns in Italy, Germany, Egypt, Russia and at the Battle of Waterloo in 1815. He took part in sixty battles four-hundred engagements and was wounded three times. He performed two-hundred amputations in a period of twenty-four hours during one campaign. He was probably the first to describe "trench foot" (in 1812), to point out the contagious nature of Egyptian ophthalmia, and he vividly described the ravages of scurvy in the French Army in Egypt. He used a flexible rubber catheter to feed a soldier who had received a wound of the glottis. His invention of the celebrated "flying ambulances" introduced a new principle in the care of the wounded during warfare. These conveyances picked up wounded soldiers as soon as the battle began, rather than waiting until the end as had been the custom previously. Stretchers of this type today are called Larreys. He originated the rule of "first aid to the wounded" in the modern sense. When the Bourbons returned to power, Larrey was deprived of his honors and attention because of his association with Napoleon, but because of his hold on the affections of the people, he suffered no bodily harm.

European medicine of the first half of the nineteenth century also contributed phrenology with its effect of stimulating investigations on the physiology of the brain; the "Irish School," and the great men of Guy's Hospital in London.

## PHRENOLOGY AND CEREBRAL PHYSIOLOGY

Contemporary with Magendie was a man whose work in Vienna had much to do with stimulating investigations on the physiology of the brain. He was Franz Joseph Gall (1759–1828) who had been trained in Vienna under van Swieten. His interest started with physiogonomy, phrenology and then cerebral physiology. His initial concept was that the talents and mental characteristics of men depend upon the function of the brain and that they can be determined by careful study of the external appearance of the skull. Johann Casper Spurzheim (1776–1832) was closely associated with Gall for several years. Gall viewed articulate speech to be located in the anterior lobes of the brain and this was confirmed and extended by Bouillaud. Phrenology became popular in all parts of the world and still exists in many cities but in the same category as astrologers and other entertainers. However, it contributed to the stimulation of legitimate investigation into the physiology of the brain and of cerebral localization.

## THE IRISH SCHOOL OF MEDICINE

During the early part of the nineteenth century a small group of men appeared in Dublin, Ireland. In that their achievements in medicine were noteworthy, they became known as the "Irish School" and included Colles, Cheyne, Graves, Stokes and Corrigan.

Abraham Colles (1773–1843) wrote the masterful paper on "Fracture of the Carpal

Extremity of the Radius" in 1814. This fracture is still known as Colles' fracture.

John Cheyne (1777–1836) was the founder of the Irish School and is best remembered for his account of Cheyne-Stokes' respiration in 1818.

William Stokes (1804–1878) collaborated with Cheyne. He also published his description of heart block in 1846. Adams had described the condition in 1827 and it has since been known as Stokes-Adams disease. Stokes' first book, *Diseases of the Chest,* was published in Dublin in 1847. This was the first modern treatise on the subject in English and considered as the best book since Laennec. His *Diseases of the Heart and Aorta* was published in Dublin in 1854. It described twenty years of his experience and contained an early, if not the earliest, account of paroxysmal tachycardia.

Robert Graves (1797–1853) described "a newly observed affection of the thyroid in females" in 1835. This condition has since been called Graves' disease and is known to be caused by hyperthyroidism. It has subsequently been learned that a similar disease was described in 1825 by Parry.

John Corrigan (1802–1880) published the *Permanent Patency of the Mouth of the Aorta of Inadequacy of the Aortic Valves* in 1832. He described the typical pulse insufficiency and this is now known as Corrigan's pulse. The article had three excellent illustrations of the appearance of the aortic valves. The eminence of the Irish School waned after the death of Corrigan.

## GUY'S HOSPITAL AND ITS GREAT MEN IN LONDON

Contemporary with the outstanding men of the Paris School and of the Irish School were the great men of Guy's Hospital in London.

Guy's Hospital opened on January 6, 1725, ten days after the death of its founder, Thomas Guy, who was a publisher and financier in London. During the eighteenth century, the hospital had excellent physicians and surgeons but no one who was outstanding. The beginning of the nineteenth century saw some remarkable men who were teachers and investigators, and were active in establishing and directing a medical school in Guy's Hospital. These men dedicated their professional lives to these activities. They had all been trained in Edinburgh and included Bright, Addison, Hodgkin and Cooper.

Richard Bright (1789–1858) pointed out the association of diseased kidneys, dropsy and albuminous urine and clearly defined the condition. It is now known as Bright's disease. He also described the frequency of cardiac hypertrophy and the increase of urea in the blood in this disease. His work was published in *Reports of Medical Cases* in London in 1827. He was better known abroad during his lifetime than any British physician of modern times.

Thomas Addison (1797–1860) described the disease in which the skin is bronze in association with disease of the adrenal glands. This was termed *melasma suprarenale* and is now known as Addison's disease. He expanded this work into a monograph in 1855 and also described idiopathic anemia. This type of anemia is now known as pernicious, or addisonian, anemia. He published the first description of the xanthoma diabeticorum in 1850. He had great skill as a clinician, a fine personality and was a leading light at Guy's Hospital during the thirty odd years of his teaching.

Thomas Hodgkin (1798–1866) described seven cases in 1832 of a disease since known as Hodgkin's disease. Later study with the microscope showed that only three of these cases are what we today understand as Hodgkin's disease. His notable work was in the field of pathology. He was a demonstrator in morbid anatomy and was curator of guy's Hospital Museum. He wrote an account of aortic insufficiency with an excellent pathological description in 1827, three years prior to Corrigan's classical paper. He described acute appendicitis clearly in his public lectures in 1836.

Sir Astley Cooper (1768–1841) of Guy's Hospital was the best-known surgeon of his time. He was trained in Edinburgh and was also a student of John Hunter in London. He became a demonstrator in anatomy at St. Thomas' Hospital and then joined the staff at Guy's Hospital as surgeon in 1800. Because of the wealth of his wife, he was able to devote himself to study and teaching but also soon became eminently successful in his own right. He was one of the best operators of his day. He successfully ligated the common carotid and external iliac arteries for aneurysms in 1808 and the abdominal aorta in 1817. He received a baronetcy in return for a successful operation for a small tumor on the head of King George IV. Cooper dissected every day of his life in laboratories which he established in his home. Existing laws made it impossible for bodies to be obtained legally and, accordingly, a macabre vocation for resurrectionists or "sack-them-up-men" developed. Because of his need for cadavers for dissection purposes, he was thrown into close touch with these "body snatchers" and became one of their main supporters. He is said to have spent hundreds of pounds on bodies and to have advanced considerable money to defend the resurrectionists when they were caught or imprisoned. He also apparently supported their families if they were imprisoned.

Cooper's books made excellent contributions to surgery and to surgical anatomy. He published *On Hernia* in 1804 and described the transversalis fascia (Cooper's fascia) and retroperitoneal hernia (Cooper's hernia). His work, *Injuries of the Joints,* was published in 1822. *Diseases of the Breast* was published in 1829, *Diseases of the Testes* in 1830 and the *Anatomy of the Thymus Gland* in 1832.

A compilation of the medical achievements of the nineteenth century will be found at the end of Chapter XVIII.

*Gentlemen, this is no humbug.*—JOHN C. WARREN, JR., M.D. (*in reference to ether anesthesia*)

# XVII American Medicine Before the Mid-Nineteenth Century

AMERICAN MEDICINE originated with the aboriginal American Indians and was developed by Spanish explorers and later by the British colonists.

## MEDICINE AMONG ABORIGINAL AMERICAN INDIANS

The time factor is important in any discussion of the American Indians. There were hundreds of tribes and they differed in language, customs and in economic, political and social organization. The Indians encountered by the Spanish explorers were different from those whom the British colonists, or Lewis and Clark, described. The Indian way of life was changed because of the Europeans, but many tribes remained relatively untouched by the influences of white civilization until the last century and a few still pursue a neolithic type of culture.

Trephining of the skull was apparently common in Peru prior to the era of Columbus and the Spanish explorers. Studies of these pre-Columbian skulls found in Peru showed that many patients survived for years after the operation. There was evidence of osteomyelitis in some of the cases with indications that they probably did not survive the procedure. It has been assumed that no anesthetic was used for these primitive procedures but in Peru the natives commonly chew Erythroxylon coca and this may have been used for its anesthetic effect. The skulls found in Peru have shown the same methods for trephining as those found in southern France from the neolithic period. These operations were performed not only for fractures, as has been determined both in Peruvian skulls as well as those found elsewhere, but for religious and magical purposes in most instances.

The early explorers and colonists who first encountered Indians were not many centuries ahead of the so-called savages from the medical viewpoint. Herbs remained the basis of *materia medica* for much of the period and theoretical concepts dominated medical thinking. The humoral theory of Galen was widely accepted in Europe and Europeans had made the major step of attributing sickness and disease to natural causes, whereas Indians looked to the supernatural. The Indians deemed that the curing of their sick or wounded was a religious duty and the medicine man represented a priestly class whose duty was to ward off the evil spirits and to summon the good ones. Trephining had no practical implications for surgery among the Indians of North America.

American Indians represented a true hunting and fishing Stone Age culture and knew only the rudiments of agriculture. They excelled in the care of wounds, fractures and dislocations because of their highly active life and extensive warfare. The aboriginal Indians had practically no experience with contagious diseases which were introduced by the white man, and which were quite deadly to them. The sweat-house was the most widely-used system of therapy for almost every malady known to the Indians. Hysteria was successfully treated by the medicine man. Snake bite was treated by suction and many tribes even excised the area. Certain Indians practiced immunization without knowing it by periodically allowing themselves to be bitten by larger and larger snakes, using a smaller one to begin with.

The medical status among the Indians was on a par with the Assyrians, Hebrews and Greeks and was of an exceptionally high standard compared to other Stone Age peoples. They handled their wounds, fractures and dislocations and empyemas as well as the eighteenth century white physician. They developed a method of removal of the retained placenta at least one hundred years before Crêde and added at least fifty-nine drugs to our pharmacopeia, including cascara sagrada.

## INTRODUCTION OF EUROPEAN MEDICINE TO AMERICA BY THE SPANISH

The Spanish were the first to colonize in America and were also the first to build hospitals and to organize medical schools. Within five years after the first voyage of Columbus they had founded the first hospital in Santo Domingo in about 1503. Cortez is known to have established a hospital in Mexico following his conquest in 1523–24. This hospital is still in operation and is known as the Jesus Nazareno.

The first universities in America were also established by the Spanish. The University of Santo Domingo was founded in 1538 and the University of Mexico in 1551. The University of Mexico created the first Chair of Medicine in 1580.

The Spanish spread their culture by means of their missions with the support of Spanish soldiers. Chroniclers who accompanied these explorers to the New World wrote vivid accounts of the land, plants, animals, people, diseases and remedies. The first medical book published in North America was produced by the Spaniards in Mexico in 1570.

## AMERICAN COLONIAL MEDICINE BEFORE THE REVOLUTIONARY WAR

The British colonists came to America to seek religious freedom and were generally of humbler stock than the Spanish grandees who came in search of glory and gold.

From 1583–1588, attempts had been made by Sir Walter Raleigh and others to found colonies on the coast of what is now North Carolina. These attempts were not successful but did stimulate the London Company to organize an expedition and to establish the first permanent English settlement in North America at Jamestown, Virginia on May 13, 1607. Disease was prevalent in this marshy low country. Colonization continued in spite of poor sanitation, summer heat, lack of food and Indian attacks. In 1619, twelve hundred new colonists appeared in Virginia and Negro slaves as well as indentured servants were imported as laborers for the first time. This same year which had witnessed the beginning of Negro slavery also saw the organization of the first representative assembly in North America, the Virginia House of Burgesses. By this time, the Virginia colonists were self-supporting and exported twenty-thousand pounds of tobacco in that year. However, the death rate was extremely high and the physicians evidently did not linger long in the colony.

The first permanent colony in Massachusetts dates from the voyage of the Mayflower which landed one hundred and two Puritans at Plymouth in 1620. Three months later, only fifty survived. Scurvy and other diseases had killed the other fifty-two.

Epidemic and other infectious diseases made the death toll high during the colonial period. Malaria, dysentery or "bloody flux" as it was then generally called, typhoid fever, influenza, as well as other respiratory diseases, scarlet fever, smallpox and yellow fever and tuberculosis were the killers of this period.

Doctor Samuel Fuller arrived with the pilgrims at Plymouth. He had lived with the pilgrims in Leyden for a period of eleven years before coming to America and may have studied at the University of Leyden. He served the colonists during the epidemics of typhus and smallpox in 1621 and visited Charlestown and Salem to help the ailing in those towns. He, himself, died of smallpox in 1633 and after his death there was no outstanding physician in Massachusetts for nearly one hundred years. After every family in the settlement of Plymouth had lost at least one of its members, the majority moved to the healthier location on which Boston now stands.

Three classes of individuals practiced what medicine there was during the early colonial period. These were the governors, the ministers and a host of minor physicians, ministers and school masters, some with medical degrees and some without. The first governor of Massachusetts was John Winthrop, who imported medicines from England in order to help the sick. John Winthrop the Younger continued this practice. The Rev. Thomas Thacher was the pastor of the Old South Church in Boston and published the only known medical publication in the seventeenth century in North America. It was his *Smallpox Manifesto* which was printed in 1677. This tract was based upon the work of Sydenham. The Rev. Cotton Mather of Boston learned about vaccination by reading of it in articles in the *Philosophical Transactions* published by the Royal Society of London. When an epidemic of smallpox broke out in Boston in 1721, he recommended it to local physicians and the first vaccination in America was apparently done in that year by Doctor Boylston. This inoculation created violent reactions on the part of the public and physicians and the practice of vaccination was slow to be accepted in America as it was where it originated.

A few qualified physicians and surgeons immigrated to the colonies from time to time but the number was insufficient to meet the needs of the steadily growing colonial population. Accordingly, young men apprenticed themselves to older physicians and went into practice without attending medical schools. There were no prescribed courses and no examination to determine the fitness of these physicians to practice. They attempted to emulate the British pattern of medicine. By the beginning of the eighteenth century, medicine in colonial America became more of a self-conscious profession and the necessity of combining the practice of medicine with another occupation declined.

The Assembly of Rhode Island and Providence Plantations conferred the first medical degree in this country on one John Cranston in 1663–1664 for his ability in comforting those who sought his skill in "Phissicke and Chirurgry." Yale College also gave an honorary degree some sixty years later to a Daniel Turner who was a London practitioner who wished to break with the barber-surgeons and to be admitted as a Fellow to the Royal College of Physicians.

The first plan on record in colonial America for the formal education of physicians was a system of lectures and demonstrations which were proposed by an Edinburgh graduate, Cadwallader Colden, in Philadelphia. However, since this plan involved paying Colden to attend the poor of the city, and defraying the cost of the establishment of the lecture series by a tax on every man older than twenty-one, the plan was not accepted. Another practitioner, Thomas Cadwalader, performed the first scientific autopsy in this country in 1742 and gave practical demonstrations in anatomy. William Hunter, who was related to John and William Hunter of London settled in Rhode Island and gave a systematic course of lectures on anatomy between 1754 and 1756. Fees were charged for each lecture and a certificate was conferred at the conclusion of the course. The first private teacher of medicine in the city of New York was Doctor John Bard.

An attempt was made to establish regulations by requiring licensure for those who wished to practice in medicine as early as 1760, when New York was the first state to enact such a law. The first medical society in the colonies was founded in Boston in 1735 and the first state medical society was that of the Medical Society of New Jersey which was established in 1766, primarily in an effort to institute licensing and to eliminate quacks.

Following the opening of the new frontier and with the developments of services for the colonists, institutions for higher learning including medical education as well as hospitals were created. Harvard College was founded in 1636 in Boston, by the Puritans, primarily to educate the clergy. Its medical school and first hospital were not established until after the War for Independence.

The Pennsylvania Hospital was established in 1751 in Philadelphia. This city had been settled by the Quakers who laid great stress on charity and was the first large hospital in North America. Its financing was made possible by the endeavors of Benjamin Franklin * and his friends. This

* Franklin has related the history of the founding of the Pennsylvania Hospital as follows: "In 1751, Doctor Thomas Bond, a particular friend of mine, conceived the idea of establishing a hospital in Philadelphia (a very beneficient design, which has been ascribed to me, but was originally his), for the reception and cure of poor sick persons, whether inhabitants of the Province or strangers. He was zealous and active in endeavoring to procure subscriptions for it, but the proposal being a novelty in America, and at first not well understood, he met with but small success.

"At length he came to me with the compliment that he found there was no such thing as carrying a public-spirited project through without my being concerned in it. 'For,' says he, 'I am often asked by those to was possibly the introduction of matching grants for the purpose of hospital construction.

The first medical school in the colonies was established at the College of Philadelphia as the medical department of the college in 1765, a short time before the outbreak of the Revolution. Philadelphia was the most influential city of the colonies of this period. Credit for founding the school is usually given to Doctor John Morgan (1735–1789) who graduated from the College of Philadelphia in 1757, studied medicine under John Redman, practiced medicine in Philadelphia in a highly successful manner, served as a military surgeon and then went to Europe to further his studies. He (Fig. 29) obtained his medical degree from Edinburgh, was admitted to many of the outstanding medical societies of Europe and, during his period of study, formulated plans for the establishment of a medical school in his native city. Morgan undoubtedly discussed these plans with many eminent physicians, including William Shippen of Philadelphia who was also studying at Edinburgh. Upon his return to the colonies, he brought with him letters from prominent members of the medical profession and from former members of the Board of Trustees of the College of Philadelphia urging the appointments of professorships for the study of medicine and surgery. The school was established with the appointment of Morgan as Profes-

←
whom I purpose subscribing, Have you consulted Franklin upon this business? And what does he think of it? And when I tell them that I have not (supposing it rather out of your line), they do not subscribe, but say they will consider of it.' I inquired into the nature and probable futility of his scheme, and receiving from him a very satisfactory explanation, I not only subscribed to it myself, but engaged heartily in the design of procuring subscriptions from others. Previously, however, to the solicitation, I endeavored to prepare the minds of the people by writing on the subject in the newspapers, which was my usual custom in such cases, but which he had omitted.

"The subscriptions afterwards were more free and generous; but beginning to flag, I saw they would be insufficient without some assistance from the Assembly, and therefore proposed to petition for it, which was done. The country members did not at first relish the project; they objected that it could only be serviceable to the city, and therefore the citizens alone should be at the expense of it; and they doubted whether the citizens themselves generally approved of it. My allegation on the contrary, that it met with such approbation as to leave no doubt as to our being able to raise two thousand pounds by voluntary donations, they considered as a most extravagant supposition, and utterly impossible.

"On this I formed my plans; and, asking leave to bring in a bill for incorporating the contributors according to the prayer of their petition, and granting them a sum of money which leave was obtained chiefly on the consideration that the House did throw the bill out if they did not like it, I drew it so as to make the important clause a conditional one, viz., 'And be it enacted, by the authority aforesaid, that when the said contributors shall have met and chosen their managers and treasurer and shall have raised by their contributions a capital stock of value, the yearly interest of which is to be applied to the accommodating of the sick-poor in the said hospital, free of charge for diet, attendance, advice and medicines, and shall make the same appear to the satisfaction of the speaker of the Assembly for the time being, that then it shall and may be lawful for the said speaker, and he is required to sign an order on the Provincial Treasurer for the payment of two thousand pounds, in two yearly payments, to the Treasurer of the said hospital, to be applied to the founding, building and finishing of the same.'

This condition carried the bill through; for the members, who had opposed the grant, and now conceived they might have the credit of being charitable without the expense, agreed to its passage; and then in soliciting subscriptions among the people we urged the conditional promise of a law as an additional motive to give since everyman's donation would be doubled; thus the clause works both ways. The subscriptions accordingly soon exceeded the requisite sum, and we claimed and received the public gift which enabled us to carry the design into execution. A convenient and handsome building was soon erected; the institution has by constant experience been found useful, and flourishes to this day; and I do not remember any of my political manoeuveres, the success of which gave me at the time more pleasure, or wherein, after thinking of it, I more easily excused myself for having made some use of cunning."

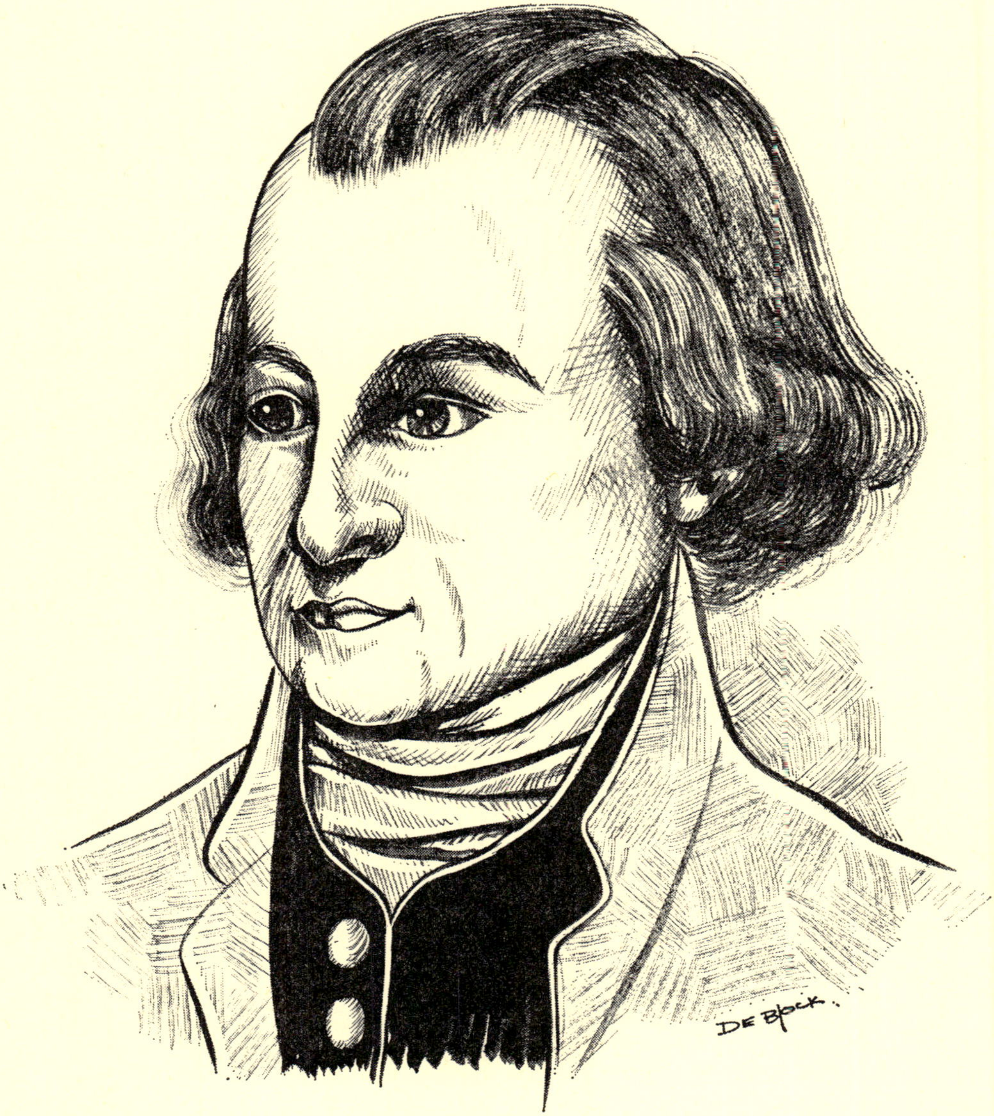


FIGURE 29. John Morgan—founder of the first medical school in the colonies.

sor of the Theory and Practice of Physic. He delivered a memorable address at the time of the establishment of the school in 1765. This lecture has become famous for its program of medical education. He had worked it out carefully while in Paris and had it reviewed by eminent critics. He pointed out the importance of a comprehensive general education preparatory to the study of medicine, the place of the hospital in the teaching program and of the eminent physicians in the city capable of receiving appointments to the faculty. He prophesied that the school would serve as an inducement for the establishment of other schools and would encourage the organization of learned societies for the spread of knowledge.

William Shippen, Jr. (1736–1808) was Morgan's contemporary and also his colleague in the establishment of the first medical school. After obtaining the best possible education in the colonies, Shippen studied medicine under his father for three years and then went abroad to study medicine under such famous men as John and William Hunter. He obtained his medical degree from Edinburgh where a medical school was discussed with Morgan. Shippen returned to Philadelphia in 1762 and began a series of lectures on obstetrics, the first course of this type to be given in America. He observed the poor quality of obstetrics practiced by unskilled old women and was able to provide beds for poor women in the Pennsylvania Hospital. He applied for and was elected Professor of Anatomy and Surgery in the new school, indicating that he had only waited to be joined by his friend, John Morgan, before proceeding with plans for the founding of the school. The first session of the new school opened on Monday, November 18, 1765, and the first class of ten students received their degrees of M.B. in 1768. Four of the ten graduates were admitted to the M.D. degree in 1771, after a period of practice and on the basis of an examination of a thesis.

Doctor Adam Kuhn (materia medica and botany) and Doctor Benjamin Rush (chemistry) were added to the faculty in 1768 and 1769. Doctor Rush was to become the most famous of all the Revolutionary-period physicians. The school grew rapidly and was well-attended. Doctor Thomas Bond (clinical medicine) was the oldest member of the faculty. Thirty-four medical degrees were conferred up until 1774, twenty-nine M.B. and five M.D.

The second medical school in the colonies was established in the city of New York in 1767 at King's College. The faculty consisted of the best men in the medical profession in New York City. The inaugural oration was given by Doctor Peter Middleton (Professor of Physiology and Pathology) who had studied at St. Andrew's University before immigrating to New York and who had, along with Doctor Samuel Bard, Sr., carried out the first "anatomy" in New York in 1750, and with him had been involved with relatives who were searching for the bodies of their deceased. The curriculum was similar to that given in Philadelphia and both schools were patterned after the European schools and particularly Edinburgh, from which so many of the faculty had graduated. The faculty included Doctor Samuel Clossy (anatomy, a graduate of Trinity College, Dublin), Doctor John Jones (surgery, also trained in Europe), Doctor Peter Middleton (physiology and pathology), Doctor James Smith (chemistry, a Leyden graduate), Doctor John Tennent (midwifery, an Edinburgh graduate and a member of the Royal Society) and Doctor Samuel Bard (theory and practice, also an Edinburgh graduate). King's College was the first school to award the M.D. degree in the colonies and also carried on the practice of awarding the M.B. first and the M.D. after an examination of the presentation of a thesis. The school was discontinued during the Revolutionary War and resumed under the name of Columbia University at the end of the war.

There were a number of contributions to the medical literature during this period and they were particularly concerned with epidemics of smallpox, yellow fever, diphtheria, fractures and numerous other condi-

*Postgraduate study has always been a characteristic feature of our profession.*—Sir William Osler

# XVIII Medicine During the Second Half of the Nineteenth Century

Paris was the unquestioned leader of medicine in the world during the first half of the nineteenth century. The second half of the century witnessed the sharing of this leadership and increasing interchange of men and scientific information.

The Industrial Age continued to develop rapidly. Japan and China were opened to trade with the West during this period with a considerable increase of markets and sources of supplies. This was the era of Queen Victoria in England, Napoleon III in France and Bismarck in Germany. The mercantile, industrial and financial worlds largely dominated European society and this middle class was strongly religious for the most part. Novelists of the day described everyday art, artists painted what they saw, musicians developed new forms and architects created functional, rather than fanciful buildings.

The nineteenth century literature was enriched by Lord Byron, Honoré Balzac, Charles Dickens, Victor Hugo, Henrik Ibsen, Sir Walter Scott, Percy Bysshe Shelley, Mark Twain and Walt Whitman. This was also the period of Monet, Renoir, Manet, Constable and Delacroix. Great composers of the nineteenth century included Johannes Brahms, Frédéric Chopin, Claude Debussy, Franz Liszt, Franz Schubert, Robert Schumann, Johann Strauss the Younger, Peter Tchaikovsky and Richard Wagner.

In America, the wealthier classes adopted the European patterns and the frontiersmen developed their own culture, based upon religion, ballad and humor. The second half of the century found itself involved in a controversy and decades of bitter debate between scientists and naturalists and churchmen. The basis of this dissension was the theory of the origin of the species and the doctrine of evolution of Charles Robert Darwin (1809–1882). However, optimism was the keynote of the second half of the nineteenth century and there was a solid belief that mankind was approaching a state of civilized respectability because of greater economic stability, more enlightened political and social reforms and the blossoming of science and technology.

The *Communist Manifesto* of Karl Marx (1818–1883) and Friedrich Engels (1820–1895) marked the advent of "scientific socialism." Its importance at the time tions. A very practical monograph, *Plain, Precise, Practical Remarks on the Treatment of the Wounds and Fractures,* was prepared by Doctor John Jones. It was widely used by American Army physicians and contained an original observation, namely, the development of hernia cerebri following trephination.

## AMERICAN MEDICINE FROM THE REVOLUTIONARY WAR TO THE CIVIL WAR

The Boston Massacre occurred on March 5, 1770, because of ill feeling between redcoats and colonists. Cold war actually existed from that time until shots were exchanged on Lexington Green in April of 1775 and the tension was, at times, intense.

Numerous physicians were prominent and influential during the formative years of the Revolution. Doctor Benjamin Rush (1746–1813) returned home from his European studies as a zealous disciple of William Cullen of Edinburgh and also of his fellow medical student, John Bostock. It was Bostock who convinced Rush of the absurdity of hereditary rulers and that no form of government is rational without the consent of the people. Rush entered the cause of American Independence and suggested the name "Common Sense" for Thomas Paine's pamphlet. He was a delegate to the Continental Congress and was one of the physician signers of the Declaration of Independence. Doctors Joseph Warren and Benjamin Church were leaders in Boston's Committee of Safety and were among the twenty-two physician members of the Massachusetts Provincial Congress.

The responsibility for a Continental Army was accepted by the Continental Congress in Philadelphia during the summer of 1775. George Washington was sent to New England as Commander and Chief and Benjamin Church, M.D., of Boston, became the first director of its "Hospital Department" at a salary of four dollars per day. Doctor Church ordered the abandonment of improvised regimental hospitals and turned several small military hospitals in the area of Cambridge and Roxbury into what was called the "General Hospital." These changes created so many complaints that an official inquiry into the functions of the hospital department in each regiment was ordered. Before these investigations were ended, Doctor Church was found to be engaged in correspondence with the British Commander in Boston, General Thomas Gage. Doctor Church was imprisoned and later banished from the country. Doctor John Morgan succeeded to the directorship in October of 1775 and inherited an almost insoluble problem. He was constantly beleaguered by meager supplies, petty politics and professional jealousy. Congress made the error of dividing the medical service into geographical areas with Doctor Morgan to be responsible east of the Hudson and Doctor Shippen to the west and in January, 1777, Doctor Shippen was named as the director general. The latter also had problems because morale in the numerous divisions of the General Hospital and at Valley Forge during the winter of 1777–1778 sunk to a new low and many army medical men disapproved of Congress' treatment of John Morgan. When Doctor Shippen resigned in January, 1781, the most violent period of the long-standing Morgan-Shippen feud ended. Shippen's successor as Director of the Hospital Department was Doctor John Cochran who served throughout the remainder of the war without being discharged or forced to resign as were his unhappy predecessors. Acute shortages and the problems of inflated currency were still present.

The annual death rate in the Continental Army from 1775–1783 was approximately 20 percent. Malnutrition, lack of medicines and supplies and poor hospital and camp conditions were responsible for the majority of the deaths, which were mainly due to typhus, dysentery, smallpox, and other contagious diseases. It has been estimated that 90 percent of the deaths which occurred during the Revolutionary War were not due to battle injuries but were the direct result of disease. It is difficult to justify the conclusion that American medicine benefited materially through the experiences of the Revolutionary War.

The medical school of Harvard College was established in 1782, one year following Cornwallis' surrender at Yorktown. Dartmouth College in Hanover, New Hampshire, established its medical school in 1798. Thus, at the close of the century, the country had four active medical schools (Pennsylvania, Columbia, Harvard and Dartmouth). These schools were intended to provide an educational experience for the great majority of American physicians at this time, but young men continued to go abroad for a medical education and, after the war, the relations with scientists and medical men abroad were resumed.

Philadelphia, New York and Boston, and eventually frontier medicine, continued to make contributions after the Revolutionary War.

## Philadelphia

Benjamin Rush (1746–1813) of Philadelphia wrote extensively and had many enthusiastic pupils. His medical theories were spread by his students and dominated medical practice for over a generation. He gave a contemporary and exact description of the devastating epidemic disease of the time in his publication, *An Account of the Bilious Remitting Yellow Fever,* which was published in 1794. Rush was a man of strong convictions and deep emotions. He advocated purging and bleeding as the major therapy in yellow fever as well as in other fevers. Rush claimed that this therapy was to reduce "convulsive action" by a process of "depletion." His *Medical Inquiries and Observations upon Diseases of the Mind* was his most important work and was published in 1812. This was the first American textbook of psychiatry and remained the only American publication in this field for seventy years. This work developed from his observation and treatment of mental patients at the Pennsylvania Hospital. He has been called the "First American Psychiatrist" because of his humane treatment of mental patients, including a good diet, exercise, hydrotherapy, his famous "tranquilizing chair" and his text.

Philip Syng Physick (1768–1837) became the Professor of Surgery at the University of Pennsylvania in 1805. He had been trained by John Hunter of London and also in Edinburgh. He and Rush were colleagues. Physick obtained a great reputation as a surgeon and teacher and has often been called the "Father of American Surgery." He introduced buckskin sutures, invented a tonsillotome, described diverticula of the rectum, devised a successful operation for artificial anus, and was the first physician in America to wash out the stomach with a tube and syringe to treat poisoning.

Samuel D. Gross (1805–1884) graduated from Jefferson Medical School in

Philadelphia in 1828 and practiced in his home city. He published his *Elements of Pathology and Anatomy* in 1839. This was the first comprehensive treatise on pathologic anatomy in the English language. He also wrote other books, including *A Practical Treatise on Foreign Bodies in the Air-Passages* in 1854. This was the first systematic treatise on that subject. He moved from Louisville to Philadelphia in 1856 to accept the position of Professor of Surgery at Jefferson Medical College. His elaborate *System of Surgery* appeared in 1870.

The American Medical Association was organized in Philadelphia in 1847. The founder was Nathan Smith Davis (1817–1904) of Chicago. The AMA published its first *Principals of Ethics* in 1847.

## New York

Following the Revolutionary War, the medical school at King's College in the city of New York changed its name to Columbia University. The medical school was not successful and the College of Physicians and Surgeons was created in its place by the regents of the University of New York in 1807. Six prominent members of the medical profession made up the faculty of the New York School. Notable among these were Doctor Samuel Bard, the professor of theory and practice and physic. Bard made an excellent description of diphtheria. David Hosack (1769–1835) was the Professor of Botany and Materia Medica. He performed the first ligation of the femoral artery for aneurysm in America.

Valentine Mott (1785–1865) was elected Professor of Surgery at Columbia University when he was twenty-six years of age and held the same appointments at Rutgers and at the College of Physicians and Surgeons. He had studied with Sir Astley Cooper, Abernathy, Cline, Sir Charles Bell, Gregory and with Monro. He was the acknowledged leader in the field of surgery for nearly half a century. He ligated the innominate artery in 1818, removed a lower jaw, excised the clavicle, ligated the common iliac artery and, according to Sir Astley Cooper, "He has performed more of the great operations than any man living." Gross stated that Mott was able to differentiate malignant and benign tumors by inspection as well as the most accomplished microscopist could with a microscope.

Austin Flint (1812–1886) became Professor of Medicine at Bellevue Medical College. He was a vigorous champion of the use of the stethoscope in diagnosis and has been termed the "American Laennec." He was educated at Harvard College and was active in founding Buffalo Medical College. He described the Flint murmur in valvular heart disease in 1862. He had great influence in his time on American medicine as a teacher and writer.

James Marion Sims (1813–1883) was Flint's contemporary. He graduated from Jefferson Medical College in Philadelphia and then located in Montgomery, Alabama. He devised an original operation for the cure of vesico-vaginal fistula in 1852. There had been no authentic cure for this condition previously. He devised the "Sims position," introduced the silver-wire suture and invented the duck-billed speculum. He located in New York in 1853 and established the State Hospital for Women. He practiced alternately on both sides of the Atlantic and is considered to be the "Founder of Gynecology" in this country.

## Boston

When the Medical School of Harvard College was established in 1783, its original faculty consisted of three men—Warren, Waterhouse and Dexter. Doctor John Warren became Professor of Anatomy and Surgery. He was the major planner of the medical school and was the foremost surgeon in New England for nearly forty years. Doctor Benjamin Waterhouse (1754–1846) was Professor of Theory and Practice of Medicine. He had trained for seven years and had been a protegé of Fothergill and a student at the University of Leyden. He was considered to be the best-educated physician in North America and helped Warren in establishing the Harvard Medical School. Waterhouse delivered the inaugural oration in Latin. He introduced smallpox vaccination in America in 1800 and crusaded for vaccination. Because he devoted so much time to obtaining a public acceptance of vaccination, he apparently neglected both his medical practice and his teaching responsibilities and became impoverished.

The third member of the founding faculty was Doctor Aaron Dexter but he left no permanent impression on medicine.

Progress in Boston during the first half of the nineteenth century was due mainly to Waterhouse's successor, Doctor James Jackson, Warren's son, Doctor John C. Warren, Jr., and Holmes.

Oliver Wendell Holmes, Sr. (1809–1872) wrote his medical classic, *Contagiousness of Puerperal Fever,* in 1843. He pointed out that the disease was frequently carried by the physician from one patient to another, or from a patient with erysipelas to a mother who had recently delivered a child. His views were vigorously attacked by the leading obstetricians of the day but history has proved he was correct. His work appeared five years before that of Semmelweiss. Holmes was also well-known as a poet and as a man of letters. He wrote *Old Ironsides* and had numerous articles in *Atlantic Monthly. The Autocrat of the Breakfast Table* was very popular in its day and it was his son, Oliver Wendell Holmes, Jr., who became the Chief Justice of the United States Supreme Court.

John C. Warren, Jr. succeeded his father as Professor of Anatomy and Surgery and the outstanding event in his professional career was the operation he performed in 1846 on a patient under the influence of ether anesthesia.

## ANESTHESIA

The discovery of ether anesthesia had a great impact on the medical world. It was received without reservation as one of the significant medical discoveries of all time and did much to bring American medicine to a maturity and equal status with the stream of medicine in the world by the middle of the nineteenth century.

Plato employed the Greek word *anaesthesia* in philosophical discussions. Dioscorides (first century) recommended mandragora to produce anesthesia before operations or cauterizations, and possibly was the first to use the term in the modern sense. The soporific sponge which Arabic medicine used a thousand years later had, as its basic ingredient, mandragora and was used to produce anesthesia. The School of Salerno also employed the soporific sponge in the ninth century and was the first to use local anesthesia in operations by means of cataplasms of hyoscyamus and mandragora. Hugo of Lucca and his pupil Theodoric wrote about the use of the soporific sponge for surgery in the thirteenth century. Ambroise Paré, Wiseman, Cheselden, Fabry, John Hunter, Larrey, Abernathy, Sir Astley Cooper, Ephraim McDowell and other well-known surgeons did not use anesthesia because of the dangers to the patient even though the early methods were described in texts on surgery in their times.

Ether was first synthesized by Valerius Cordus in 1540. Nitrous oxide was discovered by Joseph Priestley in 1772 and the exhilarating and analgesic effects of this gas were described by Sir Humphrey Davy in 1798. Michael Faraday found that ether had "effects very similar to those occasioned by nitrous oxide." Carbon dioxide was given for animal surgery in 1824 by Hickman with the production of insensitivity to pain. He asked for an investigation of his claim by the Academy of Medicine in Paris and had the support of Larrey but was outvoted and the matter was dropped.

Ether anesthesia for the purpose of alleviating the pain of surgery is distinctly a contribution of American medicine. It was used originally for the purpose of the extraction of a tooth of a patient by Doctor Elijah Pope of Rochester, New York, in January of 1842. The ether was administered by a medical student, William Clark, at Berkshire Medical College. It was the first use of ether anesthesia on record. The second use was when Doctor Crawford W. Long persuaded his patient, James Venable, to inhale ether so that Long could remove a small tumor from his neck. This was done on March 30, 1842, and the procedure was successful. Long was unquestionably the first man to employ surgical anesthesia (except for dental extractions) and he continued to use ether anesthesia for minor operations. He practiced in Jefferson, Georgia. In this small town he had no opportunity to do major procedures and his reports appeared in the *Southern Medical and Surgical Journal* in 1849.

William Morton (1819–1868) was a dentist who entered Harvard Medical School. His preceptor was Doctor Charles T. Jackson who suggested to him that the local application of ether might relieve the pain in filling teeth. This was successful and Morton then thought of ether inhalation and administered this successfully to puppies so that he could extract their teeth without pain. He was impressed by this and wrote to Doctor John C. Warren, Jr., Professor of Surgery at Harvard Medical School. He asked for permission to administer his new drug to a patient before an operation. Doctor Warren permitted him to do so on October 16, 1846. The patient was anesthetized with ether in about three minutes and Doctor Warren was able to make an incision in the neck of this patient and to remove a tumor of the jaw without any expression of pain. He was deeply impressed and became a champion of ether anesthesia. His backing played a major role in the immediate acceptance of ether anesthesia in surgery. Morton had originally called his preparation "Letheon" and planned to patent it but did not do so when he learned of Doctor Warren's opposition. Morton also petitioned Congress to grant him compensation for his discovery. By this time, Doctor Jackson had claimed the idea was his discovery and law suits ruined Jackson. Most authorities agree that Doctor Crawford Long discovered ether anesthesia but give credit to Morton and to Warren for influencing its acceptance and development as well as its introduction to the world. It is also of interest that Doctor Oliver Wendell Holmes, wrote to Morton in November of 1846 and suggested the name "anesthesia." This was adopted but it should be remembered that the same term had been employed by Plato and Dioscorides more than two thousand years previously.

## FRONTIER MEDICINE

Frontier doctors contributed notably to this chapter of the history of American medicine. Four of these remarkable men were McDowell, Dudley, Drake and Beaumont.

Ephraim McDowell (1771–1830) is known as the "Father of Ovariotomy." He studied medicine under an Edinburgh graduate, Doctor Humphreys of Stanton, Virginia, and worked as an apprentice. He, himself, studied in Edinburgh under Black, Monro, John Bell and others, but did not obtain a degree and returned to practice in Danville, Kentucky. He practiced in this town and also neighboring villages for a radius of a hundred miles or more. In connection with his practice, he was summoned to see Mrs. Jane Crawford in 1809. Mrs. Crawford had thought she was pregnant, but had sought medical help after she had passed the term of a normal gestation, and Doctor McDowell made a diagnosis of a tumor. He proposed surgery if she would come to his home in Danville. She made the trip on horseback and rested her tumor over the horn of the saddle. McDowell was able successfully to remove an ovarian tumor with the assistance of his physician nephew. This tumor weighed twenty-two and one-half pounds. He wrote a description of this condition and the operation, and also of two subsequent operations of the same kind. He sent one copy to Doctor John Bell in Edinburgh and a second to Doctor Philip Syng Physick of Philadelphia. In that Physick did not seem to be interested, he published his work elsewhere.

Benjamin Dudley (1785–1870) received his M.D. degree from the University of Pennsylvania and then spent three years with Larrey in Paris and visited Abernathy and Cooper in London. He then returned to Lexington, Kentucky at the age of twenty-nine, in order to practice surgery. He was the force behind the development of the Medical School of Transylvania University at Lexington from 1820 to 1840. He ligated the subclavian artery for axillary aneurysm and the common carotid artery for intracranial aneurysm. He published a report in 1828 on five successful cases in which he had trephined the skull for the relief of epilepsy due to pressure on the brain and was probably the first surgeon in America to perform such an operation. The new Medical College in Louisville, Kentucky was opened in 1837 and attracted most of the faculty from Lexington, except for Dudley. This exodus contributed to the end of the Medical School of Transylvania University at Lexington.

Daniel Drake (1785–1852) worked his way through medical school in Philadelphia and was unable to go abroad, but received his medical degree, after twelve years of practice. He was a forceful teacher and held eleven chairs in six medical schools during his career. His magnum opus was *Diseases of the Interior Valley of*

*North America* which he published in 1850. This was an account of the diet, habitat and occupations of people. He correlated diseases and their relationship to the topography of the country and the climate of the Mississippi Valley. Garrison reminds us that there is "nothing like this book in literature, even Hippocrates made no attempt to map out or triangulate the geographic locale of disease."

William Beaumont (1785–1853) became the first significant American physiologist. Like Dudley and Drake, he was also born in 1785. He studied medicine under Doctor Benjamin Chandler in St. Albans, Vermont, and was granted a license to practice in June of 1812, by the Medical Society of Vermont. In that year, war was declared against England at this identical time, and he joined the Army as a surgeon's mate and became post surgeon at Fort Mackinac in 1820 on the northwestern frontier. He was summoned to treat Alexis St. Martin in June of 1822 because of an accidental shotgun injury. The blast had been fired at short range and had created a hole in St. Martin's upper left abdomen of sufficient size to admit a man's fist. The wound was cleaned by Doctor Beaumont, shot as well as pieces of clothing were removed from it and the patient was dressed. It seemed inconceivable that the patient would recover, but he did. The Doctor was touched by the youth's misfortune and took him into his family, nursed him, fed him and clothed him. In that Beaumont's salary at this time was only forty dollars a month, with two to four rations daily, and he was obliged to support his family and himself, his compassion for St. Martin was evident. The boy recovered in about two years but a large fistula into his stomach remained. Beaumont conceived the idea of carrying out some experiments on St. Martin in 1825, and subsequently took the youth with him from post to post and experimented upon the gastric fluids and the process of digestion. His first four experiments were published in the *Medical Recorder* in 1826. Beaumont correctly concluded that gastric juice contains innate solvent powers and that the old theory of maceration and fermentation did not correctly explain digestion. He experimented intermittently until 1833 and St. Martin visited him periodically. Robley Dunglison, Professor of Physiology at the University of Virginia, provided chemical collaboration and Benjamin Silliman, Professor of Chemistry at Yale University found that the free acid of the gastric juice was hydrochloric acid. Beaumont's work was summarized in a book (*Experiments and Observations on the Gastric Juice and the Physiology of Digestion*) which was published in 1833 in Plattsburg and is considered to be a classic in the history of physiology.

## SUMMARY

By the middle of the nineteenth century, American medicine had come of age. Whereas, previously, it had been primitive, then Spanish and then a reflection of what was thought in London, Edinburgh, Leyden and Paris, it had now produced its own remarkable physiologists, physicians and surgeons and had taught the surgical world how to operate under anesthesia.

was slight and its basic ideas were developed later and at length in Marx's *Das Kapital* (1867–1894). This political philosophy importunes that political power passes to a politically subject group—as to the middle classes in the eighteenth century. The doctrine of class struggle leading to "socialism inevitable" was advanced. The First International Communist organization was founded by Marx with headquarters in London in 1864. It was then developed in New York. The Second International was founded in Paris in 1889. International Communism was thus established for the purpose of achieving Marxian socialism.

The Russian chemist, Demitri Mendeleyev, published his periodic classification of the elements in 1869 and the American, Thomas A. Edison built the first workable electric incandescent lamp in 1879. The technique of spectrum analysis was developed and enabled man to penetrate molecules and also the nature of the stars. The new science of anthropology was developed following the discoveries of human fossils beginning with that of the Neanderthal Skull in 1856.

Medicine shared equally in the remarkable ferment of the last half of the nineteenth century. Bacteriology was developed. Paris, Vienna, Germany, Great Britain and America were the leading centers.

## PARIS

It was the Parisian chemist, Louis Pasteur, who made possible one of the most remarkable advances of all medical history, namely, the development of bacteriology. This will be discussed later in this chapter.

New laws of electromagnetism and mechanics were applied to physiologic research and the work of the early physiologists of the first half of the nineteenth century was greatly extended by hundreds of investigators in physiology in the civilized world during the second half of the century. Claude Bernard (1813–1878) became one of the great names in physiology and certainly was the greatest physiologist in modern France. His research and concepts laid the foundations of modern physiology. He studied medicine at the Collége de France under Magendie. Under adverse conditions, he was able to discover the glycogenic function of the liver. He coined the term *internal secretion.* He demonstrated the role of the pancreatic juice in digestion. The vasomotor mechanisms were elucidated by Bernard with important studies on smooth muscle. Bernard established the basic biologic principle of homeostasis, a concept that has to do with the regulation of vital functions in the body, independent of outside factors. He termed this the *milieu intérieur.* Some of Bernard's outstanding contemporaries were Trousseau, Malgaigne, Charcot and Brown-Sequard.

Charles Edouard Brown-Sequard (1817–1894) was Bernard's successor. A brilliant, restless man, he worked not only in Paris, but in his native Mauritius as well as in London, New York, Richmond and Boston. He made three major contributions to medicine. The first was the Brown-Sequard syndrome, which he described in 1849. This is a condition in which there is a transverse hemisection of the spinal cord with loss of sensation below the lesion on the opposite side, paralysis of the extremities on the same side, and augmentation or retention of sensation on the same side below the level of the lesion. His second important discovery was the demonstration of the fact that blood vessels may be constricted by means of stimulation of the cervical sympathetics. Thirdly, he demonstrated the presence of life-preserving secretions in the adrenal glands and death with adrenalectomy. Claude Bernard had created the concept of internal secretions, but it was the work of Brown-Sequard which stimulated interest in endocrinology.

Armand Trousseau (1801–1867) was the first physician in Paris to do a tracheotomy. He was outstanding as a clinician and teacher and did original work on yellow fever and laryngeal phthisis.

Joseph F. Malgaigne (1806–1865) was an outstanding surgeon. His work on Paré included a scholarly account of the historical development of French surgery. Billings has termed him "the greatest surgical historian and critic whom the world has yet seen."

The development of the specialty of urology in the latter half of the nineteenth century, with advances in prostate surgery, renal catherization, endoscopy and cystoscopy owed much of its progress to French clinicians of the Necker Hospital. Paul Reclus, a French surgeon, introduced the infiltration method of local anesthesia after Karl Koller had discovered the anesthetic properties of cocaine in 1884.

Jean Martin Charcot (1825–1893) was one of the greatest of French teachers and clinicians. He graduated from the University of Paris and later became physician to the Salpêtriere in 1862. He lectured on chronic diseases, diseases of the aged, and diseases of the nervous system. He became Professor of Pathologic Anatomy in 1872 and was appointed to the newly established position of Professor of Nervous Diseases in 1882. Charcot created the greatest neurologic clinic of modern times and attracted students from all over the world. He was a first-class clinician, a top pathologist and neurologist and also an excellent showman.

## VIENNA

During the latter part of the nineteenth century, Vienna again became a great medical center. Three remarkable men provided the nucleus of the group which has since been designated as the New Vienna School. These individuals were Rokitansky, Skoda and Hebra. Others, such as Hyrtl, Semmelweis, Billroth, Toldt, Tandler, Zuckerlandl, Wenckebach, von Boorden, von Eiselberg and von Pirquet, were among those of first rank.

Carl Rokitansky (1804–1878) spent his entire professional life in the Pathological Institute. He performed some 59,786 autopsies during his forty-eight years of service. He made a clear and logical classification of disease from the pathological standpoint and was the first to describe, in detail, acute yellow atrophy of the liver, amyloid disease of the kidney and spondylolithesis.

Joseph Skoda (1805–1881) was one of the best-known physicians of his time. He taught that observable, physical phenomena (objective findings) are essential in physical diagnosis. He published a correlation of clinical findings with Rokitansky in 1839. Because of his skill in physical diagnosis, he became famous and also able to introduce new and better terms. He corrected certain errors made by Laennec, opposed bleeding, purges and emetics and was something of a therapeutic nihilist. It was commonplace among the more advanced physicians of this period to feel that it was sufficient to make a correct diagnosis and to have no specific treatment for the patient.

Ferdinand Hebra (1816–1880) studied skin diseases extensively in collaboration with Rokitansky and Skoda. Hebra published books on the subject in 1846, 1860 and 1876 and made the first, clear, systematic classification of skin diseases, based upon the pathology of lesions. Dermatology began a rapid development with this histologic approach of Hebra. His son, Hans, carried on in this field.

Hyrtl (1810–1895) was a scholarly anatomist of the New Vienna School.

Ignaz Semmelweis (1818–1865) became assistant in the First Obstetric Clinic at the Allgemeines Krankenhaus in 1846. This clinic, in which students came directly from the autopsy room and made vaginal examinations without washing their hands, was observed by Semmelweis to have a higher mortality rate than that of the Second Obstetric Clinic. In the latter, instruction was given to midwives and greater attention was given to personal cleanliness. Semmelweis also noted that mothers who had their children on the way to the hospital rarely suffered from infection, puerperal fever or death. He also noted that the pathological findings of a patient dying from sepsis from an infected wound were identical to those who died from puerperal fever. Thus, he became convinced that puerperal fever was due to infection and that it was transmitted to the mother by the unclean hands of the examiner. In 1847, four years after the publication by Holmes on the subject, he introduced the regulation that all examiners must first wash their hands in a solution of calcium chloride. This was unquestionably the first application of antisepsis. The point was proved by the remarkable drop in mortality to zero in one year. His concepts met with violent opposition and ridicule and probably contributed to his insanity and early death.

Theodor Billroth (1829–1894) became one of the outstanding surgeons of his time and served as Professor of Surgery for twenty-five years. He was the pioneer in the study of wound infections. His preliminary studies in this field began in 1868, one year after Lister's paper on the subject, and he then carried on his series of systematic investigations. He held that the "Cocc-bacteria septica" were responsible for wound infections and this work was published in 1874.

The New Vienna School became the mecca for young American doctors who studied abroad in the latter half of the nineteenth century, just as Paris had been previously. Laryngoscopy, rhinoscopy and the specialties of ophthalmology, otology and larynogology were all created by this School.

## GERMANY

German medicine of this period began to study nature itself, to utilize knowledge from other centers and, with the backing of a strong government under Bismarck, to develop great medical centers in a number of German universities.

Johannes Müller (1801–1858) was the pioneer of this movement in Germany and shared with Claude Bernard the reputation of being the outstanding physiologist of his time. Bernard was the last of his line, but Muller was the first of his and established a School which included some of the great names of medicine, among whom were a number of outstanding pupils, including

Schwann, Henle, du Bois-Reymond, Virchow and von Helmholtz. Müller was industrious, versatile and authored over two hundred articles. Biology, embryology, comparative anatomy, physiology, chemistry, psychology and pathology were his fields of endeavor. Müller's experiments or thoughts can be directly traced as the basis of later work by his famous pupils.

Carl Ludwig (1816–1895) was Müller's outstanding rival in physiology. Ludwig invented the kymograph in 1847. His theory that the glomerular epithelium acts as a passive filter in the secretion of urine in the kidney was advanced in 1849 and is still generally accepted. He went to Vienna in 1855 and studied the gases of the blood and described his Stromŭhr. His pupil Cloetta, with his help, discovered inosite, taurine, leucine and uric acid. Ludwig went to Leipzig in 1865 and developed a physiological institute. This center soon became a mecca for students of physiology from all lands. Ludwig also made the epochal contribution of a method of profusing organs outside of the body.

Justus Liebig (1803–1873) developed the most famous school of chemistry in the world of his time. He showed the relation between organic chemistry and physiology by means of a careful study of all material ingested and excreted. Liebig created the university laboratory of chemistry at Giessen in 1824. He discovered hippuric acid, chloral and chloroform, studied uric acid, devised a method for estimating urea, and carried out investigations on blood, fat, bile and meat juice. He introduced the concept of metabolism in his text in 1842.

Johann Schönlein (1793–1864) was the founder of modern German clinical medicine on the basis of his care in examining patients and because of his lectures. He was the first to describe peliosis rheumatica (Schŏnlein's disease) and he discovered the parasitic nature of favus.

Ernst von Bergmann (1836–1907) became Professor of Surgery at the University of Wŭrzburg in 1878 and at the University of Berlin in 1882. He was one of the finest surgeons of his time and was an early advocate of Lister's methods. Von Bergmann introduced steam sterilization in surgery in 1886 and began to employ asepsis in surgery in 1891. He advanced cranial surgery by his work on head injuries as early as 1877 and made contributions of importance on the surgery of the joints, on surgical pathology, on fat embolism and on ligations.

Theodore Schwann (1810–1882) was one of Mŭller's remarkable pupils. Schwann made one of the greatest biological discoveries of all time in 1839—the cell theory. Schleiden had discovered the same thing independently the year before, and so the cell theory is known as that of Schleiden-Schwann. This had a powerful impact on science. Cells had been seen as early as the seventeenth century by Hooke, Malpighi and others but had not been properly related to biological function. Schwann also described the sheath of the axis cylinders of nerves (sheath of Schwann), demonstrated striped muscles in the upper part of the esophagus, discovered pepsin in the stomach and showed that bile is essential for digestion.

Jacob Henle (1809–1884) actually created the science of histology. He was the first to describe that the epithelium differs in the skin, intestines, ciliated lining membranes of the surfaces, interna, tubes and cavities and included many of his own illustrations. It has been said that Henle rendered to microscopic anatomy the same service that Vesalius had done for gross anatomy.

Emil du Bois-Reymond (1818–1884) created the new science of electrophysiology with his studies on the physics of muscles and nerves. His major work was published in 1848.

Karl von Vierordt (1818–1884) published the first exact method of counting blood cells in 1852. He demonstrated a sphygmograph in 1853 and made the first tracing of the human pulse.

Hermann von Helmholtz (1821–1894), also one of Müller's pupils, possessed one of the great minds of the century. The scope of his knowledge and activities included five major areas: (1) The fundamental principle in physics of the conservation of energy. He elucidated this principle in 1846 and it has been considered to be comparable with Lavoisier's principle in chemistry of the conservation of matter. (2) The invention of the ophthalmoscope in 1851. (3) The invention of the phacoscope in 1852, in order to study the changes in the lens during accommodation, and the ophthalmometer for measuring the refractive powers of the lens. (4) The establishment of the Young-Helmholtz theory of color vision. This was based upon the color theory of Thomas Young and was developed from 1856 to 1866. (5) His fundamental work on the physics and physiology of sound which was published in 1863.

Rudolf Virchow (1821–1902) was the creator of the modern science of pathology. He (Fig. 30) is considered to have been the outstanding physician of his generation and to rank in history with Hippocrates, Galen, Morgagni, Auenbrugger and Laennec. In the field of pathology, it has been said that he was rivaled only by Morgagni but by none of his successors. The basis of this reputation is Virchow's publication of his *Cellularpathologie* in 1858. This treatise is considered to be one of the most influential works in medical history because it effectively challenged the two-thousand-year-old humoral theory. Continuing the Schleiden-Schwann cell theory, which had been elucidated twenty years previously, Virchow described the body as a community of cells in which disease was "life modified by cellular reaction against abnormal stimuli." It will be remembered that Morgagni had pointed out the importance of the pathology of an organ (and that Bichat had broken this down finer to tissues) in relation to symptoms and disease. Virchow now pointed out the fundamental role of the cell. He described many tumors and named them for the first time. His later studies on embolism, thrombosis and on endocarditis were epochal. He edited *Virchow's Archives*. He served in the Reichstag as a Liberal opponent of Bismarck from 1880 to 1893.

Julius F. Cohnheim (1839–1884) became Virchow's assistant and later Professor of Pathology at Kiel (1868–1872), Breslau (1872–1878), and Leipzig (1878–1884). Cohnheim introduced the frozen section technique for microscopic study, employed silver and gold salts for the staining of nerve endings and revolutionized pathology with his monograph on inflammation in 1873. He showed that the essential feature of inflammation is the passage of white blood cells through the walls of the capillaries and that pus cells are white blood cells which have wandered

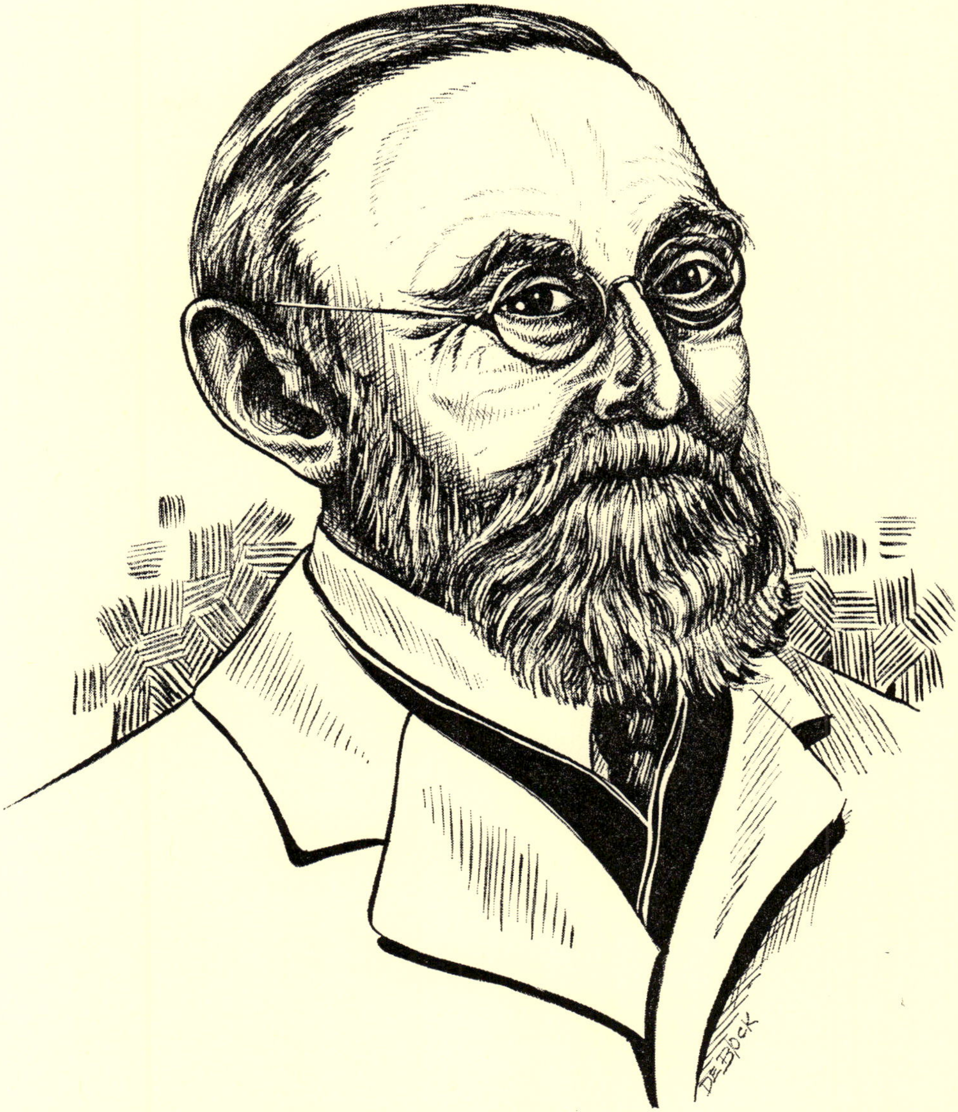


FIGURE 30. Rudolf Virchow—creator of the modern science of pathology.

from the blood cells. He was so impressed after witnessing Robert Koch's historic demonstration in 1876 of the life cycle of the anthrax bacillus, that he predicted that Koch would become the first bacteriologist of his time. Cohnheim was an inspiring teacher and had counted among his pupils such luminaries as Heidenhain, Ehrlich, Neisser, Weigert, and the Americans, Welch and Councilman.

German science made a remarkable contribution to medicine at the very end of the nineteenth century when Wilhelm C. Roentgen (1845–1923) discovered x-rays. Roentgen was Professor of Physics at the University of Würzburg at the time that this discovery was made in 1895. The way was now open for the development of the entire field of radiology. Roentgen received the Nobel Prize for physics in 1901 because of this significant contribution.

The fundamental work in bacteriology by Robert Koch and other German bacteriologists will be discussed later in this chapter under "The Rise of Bacteriology."

## GREAT BRITAIN

British medicine of this period continued its traditions of the early part of the nineteenth century and produced outstanding men and contributions to medicine. It is possible to discuss only a few of these remarkable individuals but those selected are fairly outstanding among the leaders of the era.

William Gull (1816–1890) was the leading physician in London in his time and was a worthy successor to the great men of Guy's Hospital in London.

James Paget (1814–1899) was considered to be the "foremost philosopher and orator of his day." He was the first to demonstrate trichinosis in man and did so when he was still a student. He also described two other conditions, both of which are called Paget's disease—eczema of the nipple with associated carcinoma of the breast (1874) and the bone disease, osteitis deformans (1876).

John Hughlings Jackson (1834–1911) did much to lay the foundation of localization of brain functions and to create the entire specialty of neurology. He was a leader among a group of distinguished neurologists of his time and contributed considerably to the development of the reputation of the institution in which he worked (National Hospital, Queen Square, London), described by some as the "cradle of neurology." Jackson did much to establish the value of the ophthalmoscope in the diagnosis of cerebral disease. He made important studies on aphasia in 1864 and made significant contributions to the understanding of epilepsy and cerebral physiology. Sir William R. Gowers (1845–1915) was his most distinguished pupil. Sir Victor Horsley (1857–1916) was another remarkable colleague in the National Hospital group and has been termed the "Father of Modern Neurological Surgery."

Sir Michael Foster (1836–1907) founded the University of Cambridge School of Physiology. His pupils included many distinguished scientists—Balfour, Marshall, Ray, Gaskell, Langley, Sherrington, Henry Head, Adami, Newell Martin and others. The medical historian, Garrison, has commented that Foster created "an epic in teaching that was only excelled by Ludwig's." Foster and Balfour wrote *Elements of Embryology* in 1874. Foster's *Textbook of Physiology* passed through seven editions and was translated into German, Italian and Russian.

Sir Patrick Manson (1844–1922) instigated the founding of the London School of Tropical Medicine. He demonstrated the life cycle of the Filaria bancrofti in the mosquito, and the egg of the hitherto unknown worm, the lung fluke, in the bloody sputum of a patient with hemoptysis in 1875. He retired in 1899 and continued to carry out experiments in his home with mice, rats, birds and mosquitos. He became convinced that mosquitos transmitted malaria just as they did filariasis, but was unable to prove it as there was no malaria in London. His idea, however, was passed on to Ronald Ross.

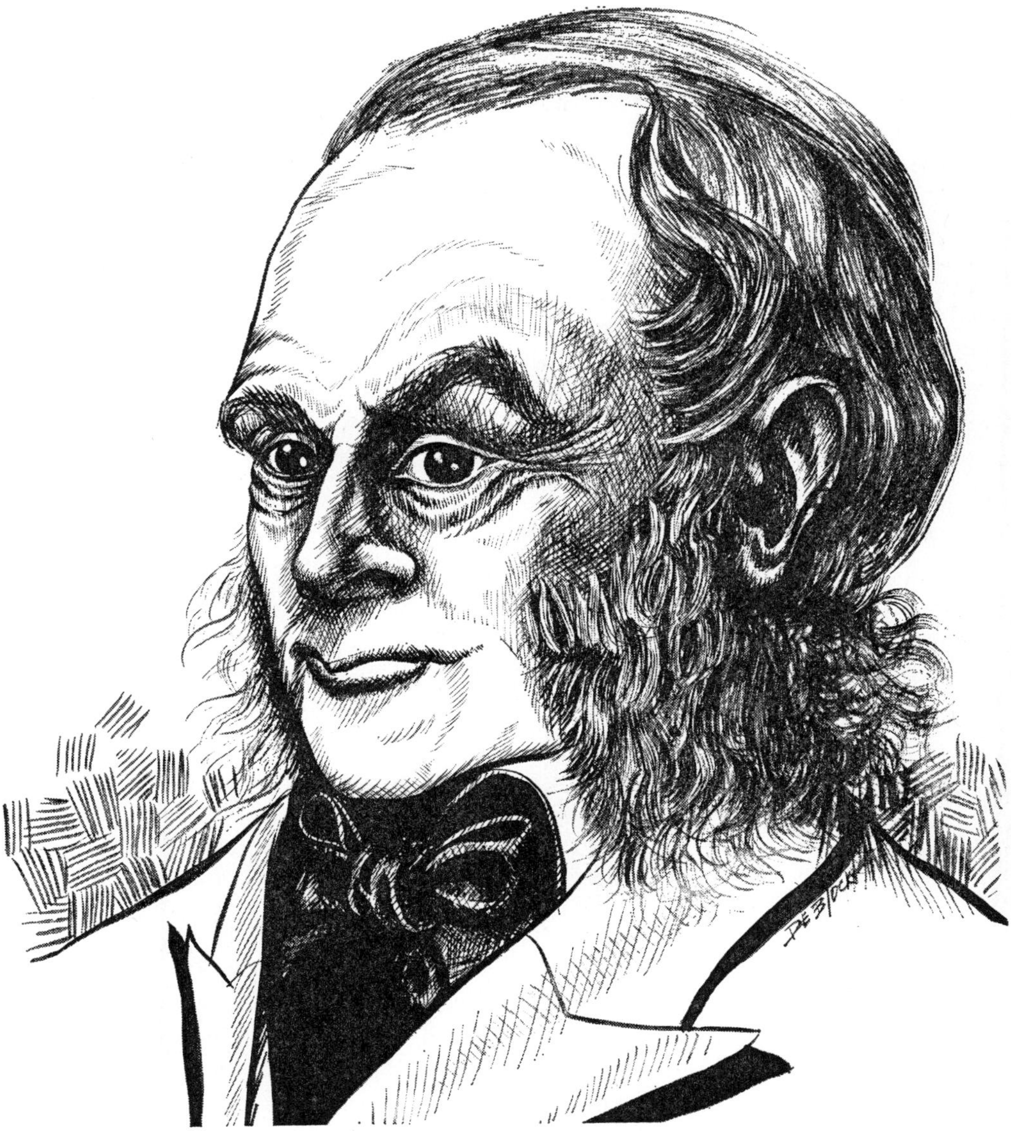


FIGURE 31. Joseph Lister—pioneer of antiseptic surgery.

James Simpson (1811–1870) was a Scottish physician who introduced ether anesthesia into the practice of obstetrics in 1847. In that ether had a disagreeable odor and a tendency to cause an irritation of the bronchi, he began to use chloroform during the same year. The clerics were opposed to this agent until it was used successfully by Queen Victoria during the birth of her eighth child in 1853. Simpson was Professor of Midwifery at the University of Edinburgh. He introduced wire suture, the long obstetrical forceps (Simpson's), acupressure (the method of arresting hemorrhage by drawing together the wound edges with needles inserted into the tissue) and dilation of the cervix of the uterus for diagnostic purposes.

Joseph Lister (1827–1912) is thought of as the discoverer of antisepsis. He (Fig. 31) was a Londoner and he received his basic medical training in London. He then went to work for Professor Syme in Edinburgh (the outstanding surgeon of Britain) and married his daughter. Lister was appointed Regius Professor of Surgery at the University of Glasgow in 1860, when he was thirty-three years of age. He taught that sepsis was the main obstacle to any great advance in surgery and concluded that air and its contents caused suppuration. This concept was based upon the observation that closed wounds would not suppurate, while those that were left open did. He was told about Pasteur's work on fermentation and putrefaction in 1865 by Doctor Thomas Anderson who was Professor of Chemistry at the University of Glasgow. Thus, the convergence of elements for successful accomplishment were again ready for a major contribution: namely, a highly trained and motivated individual, an advance in technology and a proper place in which to work. Lister chose carbolic acid as an antiseptic. This substance had been used previously in the successful treatment of sewage in Carlisle. His first striking success with the carbolic acid treatment occurred in May of 1866, although he had used it in the care of a compound fracture as early as March of 1865. He began the first use of carbolic acid spray in August of 1865 to sterilize the operative field and introduced carbolic soaked pieces of calico into the wound and carbolic dressings for the wound. After nine months of experience, he observed that he had had no cases of pyemia, erysipelas or hospital gangrene, although other wards in the hospital had their customary large number of such cases. His work was undoubtedly stimulated because of his concern at losing 45 percent of his amputation cases because of infection during his first five years as Professor of Surgery at Glasgow and his doubts on the validity of the prevailing doctrine of "laudable pus." His first papers appeared in *The Lancet* in March–July, 1867. The antiseptic method aroused bitter controversy in England but was accepted on the Continent by several distinguished surgeons, including Theodor Billroth. Ample proof of the effectiveness of antisepsis was demonstrated in the treatment of wounds in the Franco-Prussian War in 1870. Lister felt obliged to move to Edinburgh and thence to London in order to gain the acceptance of his concept in Britain. He slowly became recognized at home and abroad and became a peer of the realm with many additional honors. Certainly the dramatic development of antiseptic and aseptic surgery occurred simultaneously with the development of bacteriology.

## THE RISE OF BACTERIOLOGY

Bacteriology actually dominated the medicine of the last quarter of the nineteenth century. During the first century before Christ, Marcus Varro (116–27 B.C.) mentioned the idea that small animaliculae may cause disease. Hugo of Lucca, Theodoric and Henri de Mondeville introduced their revolutionary treatment of wounds with concern about contamination by the air in the thirteenth century but had no idea of bacteriology. Fracastoro advanced the theory that invisible living semina scattered disease. His work on infection was published in 1546 and contained the first scientific statement of the true nature of contagion, infection, disease germs and the modes of transmission of various diseases. Kircher said that he saw "innumerable small animals" in putrefying meat and "worms" in the blood of plague patients. It is not actually known what he did see and it would have required a most excellent microscope to visualize what he described. His publication, however, in 1658, was a clear statement of the germ theory of contagious disease, based upon microscopic studies. On the contrary, Leeuwenhoek, who has been described as the "Father of Protozoology and Bacteriology," sketched "little animals" but made no attempt to associate these organisms with disease. No one doubted that Leeuwenhoek saw the structures that he illustrated. His work was described in some 200 letters to the Royal Society during the latter part of the seventeenth century.

Some historians consider Agostino Bassi (1771–1856) the founder of the parasitic theory of infection. He carried out experiments at the University of Pavia and described methods of preventing muscardine of silk worms by segregation and by treatment of infected places with calcium chloride, potassium nitrate and other chemicals. He published *On Contagions* in 1844 and stated that "smallpox, spotted fever, bubonic plague and syphilis are caused by living parasites, animal or vegetable."

Jacob Henle (1809–1884) had called attention to the probability that living parasitic agents caused infectious diseases in 1840. Anthrax bacilli were seen in the blood of dead sheep in 1849 and 1850. "Monads" which were round or oval shapes were seen in the stools of patients with cholera in 1854. The term *vibrions* had also been introduced in the early years of the century for long or short moving rod-like organisms as seen under the microscope.

However, it was Louis Pasteur (1822–1895) who excited a new interest in Leeuwenhoek's "little animals." Pasteur was a chemist and his eminence in science was a result of imagination, intuition, patience, persistence and industry. Pasteur made at least six outstanding contributions to his fields of chemistry, bacteriology and industrial chemistry. His first accomplishment occurred in 1848, when he was twenty-six years of age, and had to do with the study of tartaric acid crystals under the microscope in relation to polarized light, with the demonstration of its rotatory activity to the left or right. The study of alcoholic fermentation and lactic acid fermentation in sour milk six years later led him to maintain that organisms were introduced by air and were not spontaneously generated. He demonstrated this by boiling an infusion in an open flask with the observation that putrefaction occurred. However, if the boiling was done after the flask had been hermetically sealed, the solution remained pure. This was the crucial experiment that suggested antisepsis to Lister eleven years later. Pasteur saved the French wine industry by finding that souring of wine was due to parasitic growths and that these could be destroyed by heating the wine for a few minutes at a temperature of 50 to 60 degrees Centigrade. This process was developed in 1864 and has since been extended to other fields, including the purification of milk and is known as "pasteurization." He was able to rescue the French silk industry in 1865 by the finding of silk worms feeding on damp mulberry leaves which contained innumerable "vibrions." He demonstrated that the disease could be prevented by the proper feeding of the silk worms. Unfortunately, Pasteur suffered a "stroke." He was paralyzed on his left side but recovered over a period of three months. He then resumed work and entered into the fifth phase of his major contributions, namely, that of the isolation of the microbes of anthrax in sheep and in chicken cholera and the introduction of vaccination for these diseases in homage to Jenner. His final major contribution was that of the discovery of the cause and treatment of rabies in 1885 when he was sixty-three years of age.

Pasteur's work created a wave of world-wide enthusiasm and led to the creation by his government of the Pasteur Institute in 1888. Pasteur taught that the areas of religion and science "are distinct, and woe to him who tries to let them trespass on each other in the so imperfect state of human knowledge." As a scientist he claimed absolute liberty of research. His seventieth birthday was celebrated by an international gathering at the Sorbonne. The eulogy was given by Lord Lister, following which Pasteur was presented to the Assembly by the President of France.

Meanwhile, a man twenty-one years younger than Pasteur gave bacteriology an impetus that it had never known previously. He was Koch.

Robert Koch (1843–1910) graduated in medicine from the University of Göttingen where he had been deeply influenced by Jacob Henle. Henle's theory of contagion and his importance in creating microscopic anatomy provided Koch "with both inspiration and tools to continue in an expert fashion." During the years that Pasteur was working on the disease of the silk worm and the problems of the wine industry, Koch was practicing medicine in the country. His wife bought him a microscope with her housekeeping money and Koch was able to trace the elusive anthrax bacillus through its stages by means of his methods of culturing the organism. He demonstrated his work to Cohn, Weigert and Cohnheim, as well as to other well-known scientists and they were all favorably impressed. During the following year (1877) he introduced his techniques of drying bacterial forms on cover slips, staining them with aniline dyes and photographing them for study and comparison. Because he had now advanced to the first rank in medical science he was brought to Berlin in 1878 to work in bacteriology and was given Löffler and Gaffky to work with him as his assistants. In 1881 he was successful in developing a new method of obtaining pure cultures of bacteria by using a meat infusion mixed with warm gelatin which hardened after being poured upon glass plates. Some scientists consider this to be Koch's greatest contribution to medical science because it enabled bacteriologists to obtain pure cultures of microorganisms. Using this method, he discovered the tubercle bacillus in 1882 and thus completed the long history of the search for the cause of this old disease. Koch's postulates regarding the specificity of an organism in relation to the cause of a disease were contained in his publication on tuberculosis and are as follows: (1) the microorganism must be demonstrated in every case of the disease; (2) the microorganism must be cultivated in pure culture; (3) the microorganism must be inoculated from culture to a susceptible animal and must produce the same disease, and (4) the microorganism must be recovered from the animals that have been infected by it.

Koch was able to discover the cholera vibrio in 1883 and developed tuberculin in 1890. He also found that bubonic plague was almost always transmitted by rat fleas. Emil von Behring (1854–1917) was one of Koch's students at the Berlin Institute for Infectious Disease and he became an outstanding bacteriologist. One of his major contributions was the discovery of bacterial toxins against which the body was able to form antitoxins. From this concept he was able to develop immunization for diphtheria and tetanus.

Other remarkable achievements of bacteriology during the last quarter of the nineteenth century included the discovery of the gonococcus by Neisser in 1879, the discovery of the typhoid bacillus by Eberth in 1880, the discovery of the gas bacillus by Welch and Nuttal in 1882, the demonstration of the glanders bacillus by Löffler in 1882–6, the discovery of the streptococcus of erysipelas by Fehleisen in 1883, the discovery of the diphtheria bacillus by Klebs in 1883, the demonstration of the pneumococcus (which had been seen previously by Pasteur as the cause of pneumonia) in 1884, the discovery of the tetanus bacillus by Nicholaier in 1884, the discovery of the meningococcus by Weichselbaum in 1887, the discovery of the micrococcus melitensis by Bruce in 1887, and the discovery of a plague bacillus by Kitasato and Yersin working independently in 1894.

## AMERICAN MEDICINE

American medicine had gradually emerged on the world scene by the middle of the nineteenth century as a contributor rather than as a debtor to European medicine and it continued to mature.

The American Civil War rivaled the Napoleonic wars in intensity, wide distribution of its operation and particularly in its terrible toll of men and property. General anesthesia was commonly used in operations, but modern antiseptic techniques were still to come. The majority of those wounded were injured by a soft lead musket bullet and thousands of these wounds became infected. Infections were complicated by hemorrhage which frequently caused the infection. Staphylococcus infection was regarded as a normal condition in tissue repair. However, four persons died of sickness for everyone killed in battle among those serving in the armies of the North. Diarrhea and dysentery were the major killers. Smallpox, typhoid and pneumonia were common and yellow fever and scarlet fever caused numerous deaths. Disease was also the Confederate soldiers' worst enemy and killed three soldiers for every one who died due to battle wounds. Surgeon Generals Hammond and Barnes recorded the *Medical and Surgical History of the War of the Rebellion* for the use of future army surgeons. Professional nursing service was begun during the Civil War, in order to fulfill the needs of the soldiers for care. In spite of all the difficulties of the period, public health organization, professional nursing service and a remarkably improved military medical organization were created and set the stage for future and more remarkable progress in American medicine.

Many young American physicians went to Europe and particularly to Germany for further education and then returned home imbued with the spirit of their preceptors and the institutions in which they had worked. German medicine had a tremendous influence on America in the latter part of the nineteenth century. Osler commented in 1890 in this regard:

> The Universities of Germany are her chief glory, and the greatest boon she can give us in the New World is to return our young men infected with the spirit of earnestness and with a love of thoroughness which characterizes the work done in them.

Many young men returned to America after such study and made remarkable achievements.

Henry P. Bowditch was able to establish the first well-equipped laboratory of physiology in America at Harvard in 1871. He had studied with Claude Bernard in Paris and with Carl Ludwig in Leipzig.

Reginald Fitz studied for two years with Rokitansky and Skoda in Vienna and Virchow in Berlin. He returned to Boston as Professor of Pathology at Harvard and then returned to clinical medicine. He pointed out the importance of the diseases of the appendix in 1886. His work on the appendix was one of the greatest achievements of the nineteenth century. Krönlein performed the first appendectomy for appendicitis in 1886 in Zurich.

The spirit of German medicine was particularly influential in the establishment of the new Johns Hopkins Medical School in Baltimore and this school started a new era in American medicine. Johns Hopkins University was opened in 1876, the Hospital in 1889 and the School of Medicine in 1893.

John Shaw Billings (1838–1913) had considerable influence on the plans for the organization of the new medical school and was the chief adviser of the trustees during the period of construction. He was also an adviser on the selection of the new faculty. Billings had worked for thirty years in the Surgeon General's office in Washington, was the founder of the Surgeon General's Library, an authority on military medicine and wrote the "best history of surgery that has been published in English" (Garrison). Billings traveled to Europe in 1876 to interest Daniel Coit Gilman to leave his appointment at the University of California in order to become the President of Johns Hopkins University. He then became one of Gilman's major advisers. While visiting Carl Ludwig's laboratory in Leipzig, he was very much impressed by another American and tagged him for future reference for the faculty of the School of Medicine. This young man was Welch.

William Henry Welch (1850–1934) had spent nearly two years working with Ludwig in Leipzig and with Cohnheim in Breslau. Upon his return to America, Welch established pathology as a discipline on a full-time basis in New York City at the Bellevue Medical College and remained there for a period of six years until he was appointed as Professor of Pathology at Hopkins in 1884. Welch then assumed a major role in the establishment of the medical school in 1883 and charted its course in recruitment of distinguished professors and superior students and the development of excellent facilities. His influence was great in medical education, medical research and public health and he was a medical statesman of the first rank. He became the first dean of the medical school and was also Professor of Pathology until 1916, when he became Director of the new Schools of Hygiene and Public Health at Hopkins. He

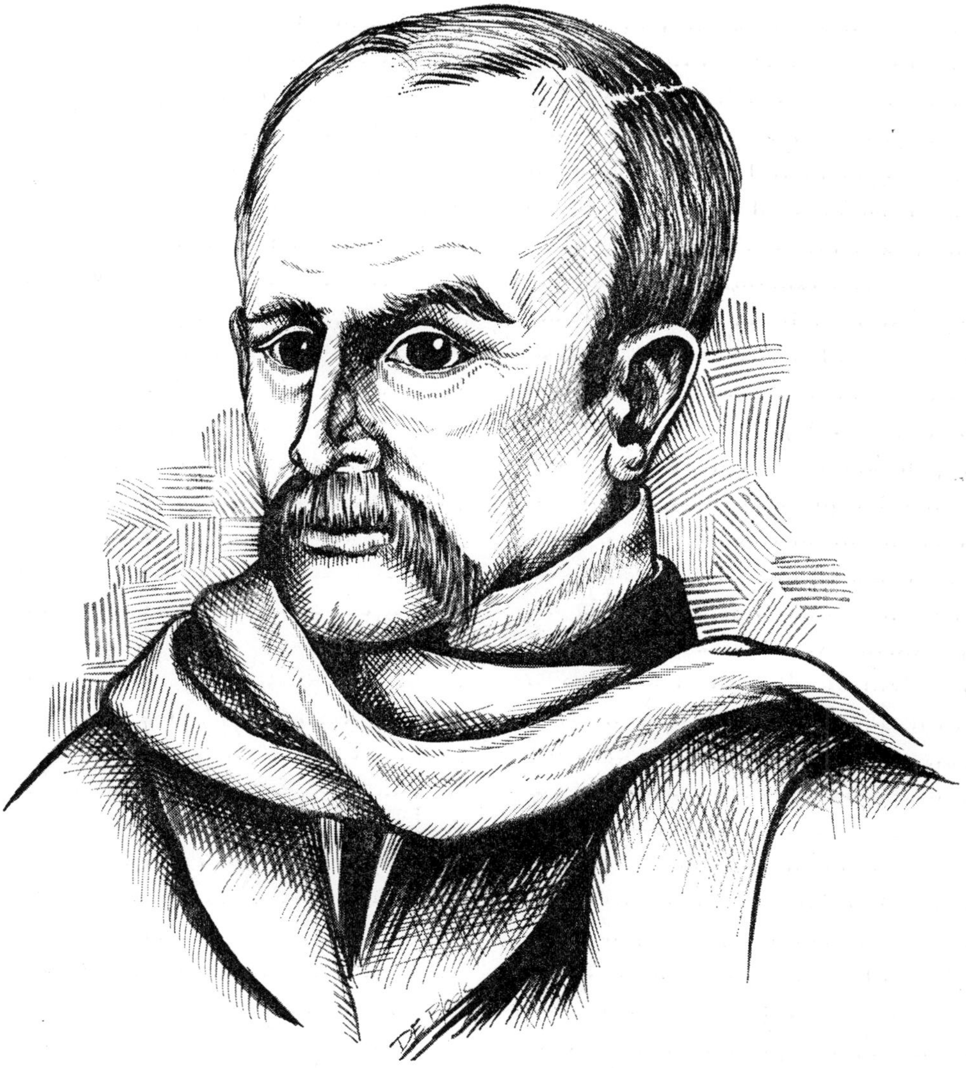

FIGURE 32. Sir William Osler—inspiring physician, teacher and writer.

was made Professor of the History of Medicine in 1926 and remained so until 1932. The William H. Welch Library and Institute of the History of Medicine at Hopkins are named for him. He established pathology in America as an independent science and specialty, discovered the well-known *Bacillus aerogenes capsulatus* (Welch's bacillus) in 1892 and the *Staphylococcus epidermidis albus*. Welch was also the architect for the organization of the Rockefeller Institute for Medical Research which was founded in 1901 and exerted a profound influence on twentieth century medicine. Walter Reed, Simon Flexner and other famous pupils were part of his legacy to medicine.

William Osler (1849–1920) became one of the most influential physicians of his generation (Fig. 32). He received his degree from the medical school of McGill University in Montreal in 1872, spent two years study in London, Berlin, Leipzig and Vienna and then returned to Montreal to become Professor of the "Institutes of Medicine" (physiology) at McGill University and pathologist to the Montreal General Hospital. He remained there for nine years and then became Professor of Clinical Medicine at the University of Pennsylvania. Upon the recommendation of Welch, he was appointed as Professor of Medicine at the newly-founded Johns Hopkins Hospital in 1889, four years before the formal opening of the School of Medicine. He introduced a combination of English and German methods of teaching and made his clinic outstanding on the American continent and a model that has since been widely imitated. Osler commented that the fate of any institution "lies in the men who work in its halls, and in the ideals which they cherish and teach." He began to write his famous textbook on medicine in 1887 and this was published five years later in 1892. Osler's *Principles and Practice of Medicine* is a recognized classic, being comprehensive, accurate, lucid, charming and warm in its style and content. The influence of Osler and his text on the medical practice of this period was great. The book had an even greater indirect influence on medical education and public health because it inspired the Rev. F. T. Gates to advise John D. Rockefeller, Sr., to enter the field of medical philanthropy and to encourage others to do so.

Two other men made up the quartet who were portrayed as "The Four Doctors" by John Singer Sargent in one of his great paintings. These two individuals, in addition to Welch and Osler, also made notable contributions to Johns Hopkins Hospital and School of Medicine as well as to American medicine during its formative period. They were Halsted and Kelly.

William Stewart Halsted (1852–1922) graduated from the College of Physicians and Surgeons in New York in 1877, interned at the New York Hospital and then spent two years abroad in Billroth's Clinic in Vienna, with von Bergmann in Würzberg and in Leipzig and Halle. He started his practice of surgery in New York City where he met Welch. He introduced the well-known "cigarette" drain for wounds in 1881 and discovered the principle of block anesthesia by the injection of cocaine into a nerve trunk in 1885. Unfortunately, his self-experimentation made him and some of his colleagues addicts to cocaine. He was cured of this by the personal care of Welch and two years later went to Baltimore at Welch's invitation to work in the pathological laboratories where he studied intestinal sutures and the thyroid gland. He became surgeon-in-chief to the Johns Hopkins Hospital in 1890 and held this position for thirty-two years. He introduced rubber gloves to surgery in 1890 and devised his well-known operations for hernia and carcinoma of the breast in 1889. The introduction of residencies as a method of graduate training for surgeons was one of his great practical achievements. This concept has now become established in the system of American medical education, not only in surgery but in all specialties of medicine. Halsted believed that competent surgeons could be trained only after years of experience under the leadership and guidance of more experienced surgeons.

Howard A. Kelly (1858–1943) was a worthy collaborator of Welch, Osler and Halsted. He was called to Johns Hopkins

School of Medicine when he was thirty-one years of age in 1889 to become Professor of Obstetrics and Gynecology. He soon became one of the leading gynecologists of his time.

## MEDICINE IN CZARIST RUSSIA

Czarist Russia had been essentially "the sleeping bear" of the world for hundreds of years. The Industrial Revolution changed the way of life in the rest of Europe and in America but not in Russia. Most of the people were serfs who farmed as their ancestors had and until 1861, could be bought and sold by their masters. Few Russians could read or write, except for the ruling class, during this period.

Peter the Great (1672–1725) forcibly introduced western habits, including military techniques, ship building, crafts and schools. He laid the basis for the Russian Academy of Sciences, ordered the children of nobility to study abroad and called in foreign professors and scientists.

The development of the natural sciences in Russia in the nineteenth century was greatly influenced by Ivan M. Sechenov (1829–1905). Pavlov, who carried on Sechenov's scientific work, called him the "Father of Russian Physiology." Sechenov attended the Military Engineering School in St. Petersburg (now Leningrad) and acquired a sound knowledge of physics and mathematics. He entered the faculty of physics and mathematics at the university and then the medical faculty of the Moscow University. He was, in this manner, provided with an all-round, natural scientific education and a good knowledge of nature, including the nature of man in all its manifestations. Moscow University had an excellent faculty by the middle of the nineteenth century and upon graduating, Sechenov was sent abroad where he spent three and one half years in various laboratories, including those of du Bois-Reymond, Ludwig, Helmholtz, Müller, Hoppe-Seyler, Bunsen, the Magnuses and Bernard. Sechenov's independent research in Russia developed under the influence of men with progressive, philosophical and social ideas. His work in the sphere of the physiology of higher nervous activity derived from his fundamental definition of the significance of the unity and interaction of organisms and their environment. His treatise, *The Reflexes of the Brain* (1863), is considered a forerunner of modern neurophysiology and the pride of Russian physiology. His work was crowned by the major discoveries and generalizations made by his pupil and follower, I. P. Pavlov. Sechenov developed the thesis that from the point of view of their origin, all acts of conscious and unconscious life are reflexes. Another fundamental achievement in Sechenov's physiological study was his fundamental conclusion that in the central nervous system there are special apparatuses, the stimulation of which leads to suppression of spinal reflexes. His concept of central inhibition was a significant advance in physiology.

Russian intellectual life continued to flourish in spite of the repressions during the nineteenth century but there was increasing dissatisfaction in spite of a few reforms. These people formed secret revolutionary societies and spread nihilist and anarchist ideas. The influence of Nikolai Lenin (1870–1924) on Russia and the world was only beginning. Russia began to expand its empire into central Asia and the

Far East during this period and to build the Trans-Siberian Railway in 1891.

## MAJOR MEDICAL ACHIEVEMENTS OF THE NINETEENTH CENTURY

Modern basic sciences and the various specialities of medicine and surgery were developed during the nineteenth century. At least six major advances were made as follows:

1. *The discovery of auscultation* by Laennec in 1816 (removing a physical diagnosis, particularly in cardiac and pulmonary disease, from the realm of speculation to the field of demonstrated fact).
2. *The discovery of ether anesthesia* for general surgery by Long in 1842 and Morton in 1846 (thus permitting the patient and surgeon to regard surgery with more equanimity and for the science of surgery to advance with rapidity).
3. *The cellular theory of Virchow* which was published in his *Cellularpathologie* in 1858 (introducing a new medical concept and destroying the erroneous humoral theory of health and disease which had dominated medicine for two-thousand years).
4. *The development of the science of bacteriology* by the discoveries of Pasteur, Koch and their pupils (thus making possible the discoveries of the causes of many diseases and new methods of prevention, control and cure of these diseases).
5. *The development of antiseptic surgery* by Lister in 1867 and of *aseptic surgery* by von Bergmann in 1891, which made it safer to operate and to reduce remarkably the previously high mortality rate.
6. *The discovery of "x-rays"* in medicine by Roentgen in 1895, which added further precision to diagnosis in various diseases and was the beginning of the specialty of radiology.

*The keynote of progress in the twentieth century is system and organization—in other words, "team work."*—DOCTOR CHARLES H. MAYO

# XIX Twentieth Century Medicine

THE WORLD about 1900 seemed to be at the height of modern imperialism. The European or Western powers and one non-Western state, Japan, dominated the other parts of the world and most of Asia, Africa and the Pacific Islands were under colonial rule. The greatest of colonial empires was the British and it was held together by British trade, British capital, the British Islands and the British Navy whose supremacy no one contested. Unlike the others, the Russian Empire spread across the land mass contiguous to it's own home country. France had lost a colonial empire in the eighteenth century and had acquired another during the nineteenth century, mostly in Africa, Indo-China and various Pacific Islands. Germany, Italy, Belgium, the United States, Japan and the Dutch were all involved in the colonial field. This state of affairs remained essentially unchanged until World War I.

In connection with the development of worldwide interest in business, industry and science, enormous personal fortunes were created on both sides of the Atlantic Ocean. Two of these captains of industry are particularly remarkable not only for their direct influence on the development of twentieth century medicine and science, but also because of their example and encouragement for philanthropists and governments to support such endeavors. These individuals were Alfred Nobel and John D. Rockefeller. They, and other men like them, actually surpassed the Medicis and other patrons of the Renaissance in their philanthropy.

## ROCKEFELLER AND THE ROCKEFELLER INSTITUTE

John D. Rockefeller (1839–1937) made his fortune in the oil business and at one time was supposedly the world's richest man. He was a thinker, planner, entrepreneur and, most of all, a philanthropist. He was the son of a peddler and started to work at the age of sixteen as a clerk in a small produce firm. He became a partner in a grain commission house and then entered the oil business at the age of twenty-three. He was able to bring the control of oil production and refining under one company during a period of fifteen years. The vastness of his holdings, and public criticism of his competitive methods, caused the courts to dissolve the Standard Oil Trust in 1892 and a holding company, Standard Oil Company of New Jersey, took its place. Rockefeller retired from active management of the business in 1894–1895 and even before his retirement devoted a large part of his efforts to his many philanthropies. From 1895 until his death, he spent most of his time in planning and establishing the foundation through which he gave his money to the public. He gave away well over 500 million dollars before his death and most of this went to foundations and organizations. The best known of his foundations are the Rockefeller Foundation, the Rockefeller Institute, the General Education Board and the Laura Spellman Rockefeller Memorial.

The Rockefeller Institute for Medical Research was the beginning of a new era in American and world medicine. The Rev. Frederick T. Gates, a Baptist minister who, in his later years, became one of Rockefeller's philanthropic advisers, had read Osler's remarkable text, *Principles and Practice of Medicine,* which was published in 1892. He apparently was much impressed by Osler's book and also the fact that, in Osler's opinion, only four or five diseases were actually subject to medical cure. After reading this book during his summer vacation in 1897, Gates called Mr. Rockefeller's attention to this state of affairs and also to the Pasteur Institute in Paris and the Koch Institute in Berlin. Rockefeller took the matter up with his son, John D. Jr., who continued this interest and an interest in medicine throughout his life. Conferences were held with leading medical men and Doctor William Welch of Johns Hopkins was made chairman of the Scientific Advisory Board and delegated to create an institute. The Rockefeller Institute for Medical Research was planned largely by Doctor Welch and was founded in 1901. One of Welch's pupils, Doctor Simon Flexner, was selected as the first director. At first, the Institute gave grants-in-aid to research in other institutions, but temporary laboratories were opened in 1904 and in 1906 the Institute was established at its present location on the East River. William Welch became president of the board of directors and remained so for a period of thirty-years. The Rockefeller Hospital was completed in 1910 and was the first hospital in America to be devoted entirely to clinical investigations. The Rockefeller Institute became to the public and to the medical profession alike what the Pasteur Institute was to France; it has made notable contributions in chemistry, infectious diseases, parasitology, tumor research, virus disease and has provided a number of Nobel Prize winners. The *Journal of Experimental Medicine* was taken over by the Rockefeller Institute and immediately became productive in furnishing the profession with a steady flow of scientific articles about many fields of medicine. Rockefeller had also given 35 million dollars to the founding and support of the University of Chicago before 1910. The Rockefeller Foundation was created in 1913 and served broad fields on a worldwide basis. The General Education Board provided a gift of 1½ million dollars to Johns Hopkins University so that the full time faculty system could be established in 1914. The Rockefeller Institute and Hospital have had many luminaries, in addition to William Welch and Simon Flexner, including S. J. Meltzer (founder of the Society of Biology in Medicine and its journal), Abraham Flexner (author in 1910 of the *Carnegie Report* * which created the beginning of a

* The Carnegie Foundation for the Advancement of Teaching had decided to use part of the income

new era for medical schools in this country), Alexis Carrel (pioneer in vascular surgery and organ transplantation), Donald Van Slyke (outstanding clinical chemist), Karl Landsteiner (authority on the mechanism of immunity and the man who introduced blood grouping), and Peyton Rous (Nobel Prize-winning cancer research scientist). George Vincent, Alan Gregg, Detlev Bronk and others have similarly exerted enlightened leadership for the Rockefeller Foundation.

The Rockefeller Institute has had more than a passing influence in stimulating other wealthy men to invest in health. Nuffield, Wellcome, Carnegie, McCormick, Phipps, Mellon, Ford, Kresge, Macy, Cullen, Whitney, the duPonts, Hughes, to name a few, have made significant contributions to twentieth century medicine.

## NOBEL AND HIS PRIZES

Alfred Bernhard Nobel (1833–1896) was a Swedish chemist who invented dynamite and also founded the Nobel Prizes. He was born in Stockholm, Sweden. His father was an engineer and an inventor. He was educated in St. Petersburg, Russia and later studied engineering in the United States. Nobel experimented with nitroglycerin in his father's factory and hoped to make this substance into a safe and useful explosive. So many accidents occurred when it was put on the market that he was considered to be a menace to society. In 1867, Nobel combined nitroglycerin with kiselgühr as *dynamite* and this explosive could be handled and shipped safely. He set up factories throughout the world, took out three hundred fifty-five patents on various inventions and amassed a fortune from them and from the oil fields in Baku. He became one of the world's richest men. He also worked on artificial silk, synthetic rubber and many other patented products, was fond of literature and wrote several plays and novels. His will created a fund which amounted to nine million dollars and was explicit in its provisions. The earnings from this capital were designated to be distributed in the form of prizes "to those who during the preceding year shall have conferred the greatest benefit on mankind."

### Alfred Nobel's Will

The whole of my remaining realizable estate shall be dealt with in the following way:

The capital shall be invested by my executors in safe securities and shall constitute a fund, the interest on which shall be annually distributed in the form of prizes to those who, during the preceding year, shall have conferred the greatest benefit on mankind. The said interest shall be divided into five equal parts, which shall be apportioned as follows: one part to the person who shall have made the most important discovery or invention within the field of physics; one part to the person who shall have made the most chemically important discovery or improvement; one part to the person who shall have made the most important discovery within the domain of physiology or medicine; one part to the person who shall have produced in the field of literature the most outstanding work of idealistic tendency; and one part to the person who shall have done the most or the best work for fraternity among nations, for the abolition or reduction of standing armies and for the holding and promotion of peace congresses.

The prizes for physics and chemistry shall be awarded by the Swedish Academy of Science:

← of the Fund for Educational Inquiry to study the education for the learned professions. Henry Pritchett, the first president of the Foundation, met with no encouragement for this study from organized theology or law but the American Medical Association and its president, Doctor William Welch, discovered great mutual interest and the report of Flexner was initiated.

that for physiological or medical works by the Caroline Institute in Stockholm; that for literature by the Academy in Stockholm; and that for champions of peace by a committee of five persons to be elected by the Norwegian Storting. It is my express wish that in awarding the prizes, no consideration whatever shall be given to the nationalities of the candidates, so that the most worthy shall receive the prize, whether he be a Scandinavian or not.

*Paris, November 27, 1895*

ALFRED BERNHARD NOBEL

Winners are chosen in November and the awards are made on December 10, on the anniversary of Nobel's death in 1896. The prizes are presented by the King of Sweden in the Stockholm Concert Hall. The Nobel Prize is currently worth approximately 40,000 dollars (tax free). The Nobel laureates in medicine and physiology are the recipients of a gold medal (Fig. 33) and a diploma which is a citation of the achievements of the awardee.

In many respects, the history of the Nobel laureates in medicine and physiology reflects the progress of medicine during the twentieth century. Americans have won the majority of the Nobel Prizes in the fields of physics, physiology and medicine and peace. The British are next and the Germans a close third in the field of physics. The Germans lead in chemistry and the French in literature.

Evolution of twentieth century medicine is represented by three generations or eras, namely: (1) to World War I, (2) between World Wars I and II, and (3) since World War II. As usual, there is considerable interlacing and overlapping of individuals and events from era to era. The mass of data is quite overpowering and, in that the author's medical life began in 1936 on admission to medical school, balanced judgment as to what is permanent and what is of passing value since then is more difficult than with previous periods of time.

## MEDICINE TO WORLD WAR I

The discoveries of the twentieth century would not have been possible without those of the nineteenth and preceding centuries. Important advances in chemistry, bacteriology, pathology, physiology, physics and pharmacology made the opening years of the twentieth century truly the golden age of German medicine.

Bacteriology continued to develop rapidly. Löffler had already detected ultramicroscopic organisms with the use of the ultramicroscopic filter in 1898 in the Imperial Health Office in Berlin. He found types of filterable viruses, including those causing smallpox, cowpox, influenza and many others in these same laboratories where Koch and others had made such epochal discoveries previously. An outstanding contribution to medicine was made by Fritz Schaudinn, (1871–1906) when he discovered that the *Spirochaeta pallida* was the cause of syphilis. The cause of syphilis had been sought for more than twenty years by numerous bacteriologists and many false claims had been made previously. The discovery by Schaudinn ranks with Koch's discovery of the tubercle bacillus and opened the new era in the study of syphilis. His work was done in 1905. August von Wassermann (1866–1925) discovered the Wassermann reaction for syphilis in 1906. These remarkable discoveries stimulated other studies related to the problems of syphilis. Paul Ehrlich (1854–1915) was one of the outstanding medical scientists of this period and when a special institute was established for him in

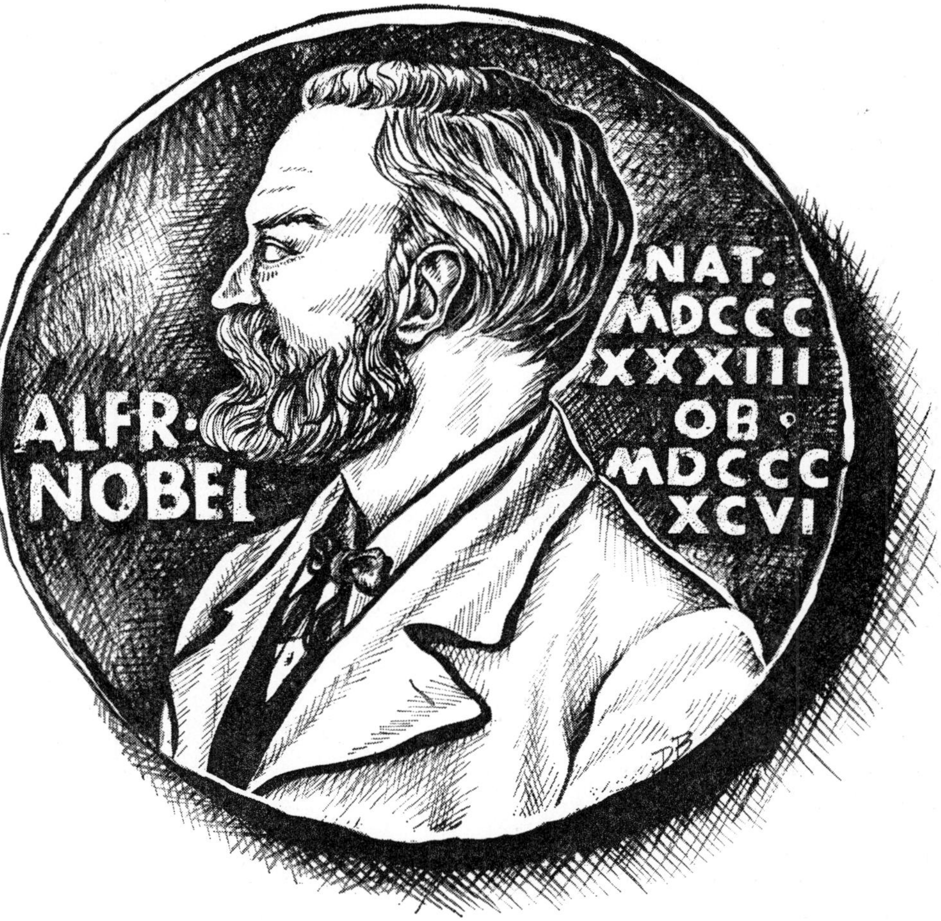


FIGURE 33. The Nobel Prize—gold medallion.

1906, he realized his long ambition of devoting himself entirely to the systematic study of chemotherapy. His outstanding work was that on the effects of arsenical compounds in experimental syphilis and his discovery of salvarsan (compound 606) occurred in 1910. Ehrlich had dreamed of complete sterilization of infection with salvarsan but this did not materialize. The preparation was used for a generation as the most potent and widely-used drug in the treatment of syphilis. Ehrlich had demonstrated near the end of the nineteenth century, specific staining of the granules in white blood cells. He received the Nobel Prize in medicine in 1908 as the father of modern chemotherapy and hematology.

A significant advance in bacteriology was made by a United States Army Board, headed by Major Walter Reed in 1900, when this group demonstrated that either an ultramicroscopic organism or a filterable virus is transmitted to man by a particular species of mosquito, the *Aedes aegypti*, in order to cause yellow fever. This work is considered to be among the most brilliant and conclusive in the history of science and made it possible to eradicate yellow fever in the United States, the West Indies and the rest of the world. The Panama Canal became feasible because of this new ability to control yellow fever.

German chemistry also continued to advance and Emil Fischer (1852–1919) carried on in the traditions of Liebig, Wöhler and Kekulé. He synthesized proteins from amino acids, discovered a host of chemical compounds, synthesized purines, caffeine, xanthine and theobromines and clarified the relationship of these purine compounds to gout. He produced polypeptides, demonstrated enzymes, synthesized veronal and thus initiated work on barbiturates. He received the Nobel Prize in chemistry in 1902.

Medical clinics in Germany were models for the world in their teaching methods and in the availability of clinical material. The Second Medical Clinic in Münich was directed by Friedrich von Müller who has been described by Garrison (1912) as "perhaps the most scientific teacher in Internal Medicine today." Abraham Flexner wrote in 1912 of this clinic in the following way:

> The professor reads the history, displays on the blackboard the temperature chart, then in quick, clear fashion explores the patient, pointing out what he finds, discoursing on its significance, suggesting alternate explanations . . . the etiology, the pathology, the therapeutics . . . of the conditions are set forth with wonderful vigor and rapidity . . . A master-mind at work is exhibited daily to two hundred students or more.

Science had no way of measuring nutrition before the time of von Müller. He conceived the idea of a unit of measurement and called it a "calorie." Müller found that a gram of fat yielded 9.12 calories, a gram of carbohydrate, 4.1 calories and a gram of protein, 4.1 calories. This discovery made possible the scientific feeding of patients with diabetes mellitus, obesity, inanition and opened the specialty of dietetics.

Karl Sudhoff (1853–1938) who established the Institute of Medical History in Leipzig in 1905 was a classical scholar and medical practitioner. He founded the *Archives for the History of Medicine* in 1908 and published on the history of dentistry, the School of Salerno and a number of other subjects. He is considered by Major to have been the greatest medical historian of modern times. His pupils have been active in major medical centers of the world in the field of medical history.

The surgical clinics in Germany equaled those in medicine. August Bier was a Professor of Surgery in Berlin. He made the first successful clinical use of spinal anesthesia in 1898 and was one of many outstanding surgeons in Germany.

German-speaking Vienna was one of the most active centers for medical teaching and research in the world at this time. American medical students came to Vienna in such numbers that they founded the American Medical Association of Vienna. The faculty consisted of Carl Norden in metabolic diseases, Wenckebach in cardiology, Chvostek and others in internal medicine, von Pirquet and Schick with their skin tests for tuberculosis and diphtheria, von Eiselberg (Billroth's pupil) in surgery, Lorenz in orthopedic surgery, Weichselbaum in pathology, Toldt in anatomy, Neuburger in medical history, von Jauregg and Sigmund Freud in psychiatry and others.

One of the greatest physiologists of modern times was a Russian, Ivan Petrovich Pavlov (1849–1936). A pupil of Sechenov, the Russian physiologist, he also studied with Heidenhain in Breslau and with Ludwig in Leipzig. He then returned to St. Petersburg in the department of physiology at the Army Medical Academy and became the director of the Institute of Experimental Medicine in 1890. His work was only temporarily interrupted by the Russian Revolution and he continued as an honored scientist under the Communist regime. His two outstanding contributions to medicine were (1) the relationship of psychic stimuli to digestion, and (2) the discovery of conditioned reflexes. Pavlov received the Nobel Prize in 1904 for his epochal studies on digestion.

The Nobel Prizewinner of medicine in 1906 was Santiago Ramón y Cajal (1852–1934) for his pioneer work in the study of the finer anatomy of the nervous system. He is one of the few medical men from Spain to achieve international reputation. The Spanish people and their government had been reluctant to support medical research and medical education because of other interests and Cajal, like others in his country, worked against great odds. He eventually was so recognized that in his later years the Ramón y Cajal Institute was constructed in Madrid for his work in the study of the finer anatomy of the nervous system and became a mecca for students and specialists in this area of medicine.

One of the great masters of surgery in the early part of the twentieth century was Theodor Kocher (1841–1917) whose entire life and career were spent in Bern, Switzerland. His major contributions were his work on the problems of goiter, colloid and toxic. He received the Nobel Prize in medicine in 1909 because of his well-known investigations in this field. His influence on surgeons, young and old, was immense. He studied surgical problems in the operating rooms and in the physiological and pathological laboratories. He investigated intracranial pressure, bullet wounds and lesions of the spinal cord. His skill and perfect aseptic technique were remarkable. His American contemporary, Halsted, admired Kocher and resembled the Swiss surgeon in many ways. Kocher had great influence on Halsted's pupil, Harvey Cushing, and they collaborated in Bern on fundamental studies on intracranial pressure when Cushing was thirty-one years of age. Cushing's first impressions of Kocher's clinic were recorded in his diary for November 1, 1900 as follows:

> Kocher's clinic in A.M.—But the operating!—the Johns Hopkins Hospital outdone. It's easy to see why "the Professor" thought so highly of their work. Detailed technique, tedious operating, absolute hemostasis.

Rickettsial diseases were discovered in the early years of the twentieth century. Small bacilli transmitted by ticks and lice to human beings were found to be the causative organisms. Five or more diseases are now recognized as being due to this distinct type of microorganism and have been named for Howard T. Ricketts (1871–1910) who lost his life due to Mexican typhus when he was thirty-nine. He was able to link infected ticks to the cause of Rocky Mountain spotted fever in 1906. Von Prowazek associated lice with typhus fever in 1913. Rickettsial diseases include typhus fever, Rocky Mountain spotted fever, trench fever, Mexican typhus, Japanese river fever and Q fever.

Knowledge about vitamins developed as an achievement of the twentieth century for the most part. Lind's, *A Treatise of the*

*Scurvy,* which was published in 1753, instituted the beginning of our knowledge of vitamins, and a daily ration of lemon juice to the sailors of the British Navy during a twenty-three week voyage in 1794 was the first practical treatment. Christian Eijkman published about the similarity between beri-beri and a polyneuritis in chickens in 1890. He found that these conditions could be produced by feeding chickens polished rice and cured by either feeding them unpolished rice or treating them with aqueous or alcoholic extracts of the polishings. Gowland Hopkins demonstrated that rats failed to grow on a diet of artificial milk but gained weight and grew rapidly when a small quantity of cow's milk was added daily. He concluded that there must be some additional substances in food which he called "accessory substances," or "indispensable ingredients in the food." It was he who suggested that the accessory substance in lemon juice was the indispensable ingredient to prevent scurvy. His experiments on feeding rats were done in 1906. Casimir Funk published his *The Etiology of Deficiency Diseases* in 1912 and described how yeast would cure or prevent beri-beri. He proposed that the substance essential for life and growth was an amine and suggested the name "vitamine" for the accessory substance. When it was determined later on that these substances were not amines the name was changed to *vitamin.* A vast literature on the development concerning various vitamins developed during the early years of the twentieth century and specific vitamins became associated with night blindness, beri-beri, scurvy, rickets, pellagra and other conditions. Hopkins and Eijkman shared the Nobel Prize in medicine in 1929 for their contribution to this work. This prize was also awarded in 1927 to Albert Zent-Gyorgyi for isolating vitamins C and P and in 1940 to Henrick Dam for isolating vitamin K.

The role of allergy in disease was another achievement of the early years of the twentieth century. Allergic symptoms had been described by Rhazes (865–925 A.D.) in patients who had sneezing and itching of the nose whenever they came in contact with roses, and van Helmont (seventeenth century) described attacks of asthma caused by house dust and by eating fish which was fried in oil. John Bostock wrote on "summer catarrh" in 1819 and Morrill Wyman demonstrated on himself that hay fever could be induced by sniffing ragweed pollen.

However, it was Charles Richet, a French physiologist, whose investigations clarified the reasons for allergic phenomena. Working in 1902 with toxin from the Portuguese man-of-war jelly fish, he observed that this could cause urticaria (hives) on contact, that a single injection of this toxin into an animal might produce no effect and that a second injection of the same toxin could be fatal a few days later. He called this phenomena *anaphylaxis,* which means "a lifting up or removal of protection" as compared with *prophylaxis,* which means "favoring protection." Richet was awarded the Nobel Prize in medicine in 1913 for this work. The term *allergy* was suggested by von Pirquet for the Richet phenomena of anaphylaxis. Allergy means a changed state rather than just diminution of protection. Von Pirquet's skin test for tuberculosis was regarded by him to represent an allergy to the tubercle bacillus. Meltzer pointed out that asthma might be an allergic process and that allergy may cause skin diseases and be a factor in the morbidity and mortality in some infectious diseases. Meltzer carried out his work at the Rockefeller Institute in 1910. Allergy has continued to develop and has become one of the important specialties of internal medicine.

Ludwig Aschoff (1866–1942) was the preeminent pathologist of his day and the discoverer of a new anatomical system of body cells, the reticuloendothelial system. As successor to Virchow and Cohnhein, Aschoff found that the reticuloendothelial system played an important role in health and in certain rare diseases associated with lipoid. He created the largest school of pathology of his day but his career was interrupted and ruined to a large extent by World War I.

Developments in physics proved to be of extreme value to medicine near the turn of the century. Discoveries of radium and of the string galvanometer were outstanding in this regard.

Radium was discovered by Pierre and Marie Curie and was announced to the French Academy of Sciences by Henri Becquerel in 1898. Becquerel was the French physicist who had asked the Curies to investigate his observation that a piece of uranium ore affected a photographic plate. The finding of an element which possessed radioactivity led to its use in the treatment of certain diseases which could not be safely treated by means of x-ray therapy.

The string galvanometer was made in 1903 by William Einthoven who was Professor of Physiology at the University of Leyden. Einthoven also made the first electrocardiograph and this gave clear records of the electrical changes in the beating heart and opened a new era for cardiovascular medicine. He received the Nobel Prize in medicine in 1924 as the inventor of the electrocardiograph. Doctor James Herrick of Chicago emphasized the role of occlusion of the coronary arteries in myocardial infarction and Sir Thomas Lewis of London enhanced our knowledge of the circulation and its diseases. Coronary occlusion was described for the first time by Doctor James B. Herrick, of Chicago, in 1912.

Cardiology was further advanced by Sir James Mackenzie (1853–1925). He published his *The Study of the Pulse* in 1902 and his *Diseases of the Heart* in 1908. He devised an ingenious polygraph to record pulse irregularities. The contributions by Einthoven and Mackenzie are considered to represent the first major advance in cardiology since the discovery of auscultation by Laennec.

Many very noteworthy physicians worked in various parts of the world during the first part of the twentieth century and it is not possible to do justice to all of them in this presentation. A few of these remarkable individuals have been selected to represent their many colleagues.

Sir Jonathan Hutchinson was knighted for his distinguished services to medicine in 1908. Few medical men have been so versatile. Syphilis interested him and it is said that he saw more than a million patients suffering from this disease. He is best remembered for his description of a certain deformity of teeth characteristic of hereditary syphilis.

Sir Ronald Ross discovered malarial parasites in the stomach of the anopheles mosquito and proved the role of the mosquito in the transmission of malaria in 1897. He received the Nobel Prize in medicine in 1902 for this achievement.

Harvey Cushing (1869–1939) established neurological surgery as a full-time specialty. He graduated from Harvard

Medical School in 1895, was trained in surgery by Halsted and inspired as a scholar by Osler at Johns Hopkins. His *The Pituitary Body and its Disorders* was published in 1912 and was a surgical and physiological classic which did much for the further development of endocrinology. He and his school, Percival Bailey, Walter Dandy, Wilder Penfield and other remarkable men, are largely responsible for the development of modern neurological surgery.

Sir Henry Head (1861–1940) was England's leading neurologist during the early years of the twentieth century. He studied at Cambridge under Michael Foster, W. G. Haskell and J. N. Langley. His first publication, *Disturbances in Sensation with Special Reference to the Pain of Visceral Disease* in 1893, became a milestone in neurology and recognized the existence of referred pain and established the painful areas on the surface associated with disease of organs. He also provided a classical work, *Aphasia and Kindred Disorders of Speech* (two volumes), in 1926.

The psychiatrist of 1900 was better able to classify psychoses and to predict their outcome than had been his predecessors a century before, but he still was ignorant of the causes of mental disease and offered mainly custodial care. Sigmund Freud (1856–1939) became the most celebrated psychiatrist during the first half of the twentieth century. His ideas developed into an international movement and became the basis for psychoanalysis. He began to study dreams in order to interpret neuroses, recognizing that the basic force in therapy was the phenomena of transference with an element of suggestion. The International Psychoanalytic Association was founded in 1910 by Freud, Bleuler, Jung and Ferenczi. Two of his most gifted pupils, Alfred Adler and C. G. Jung left him in 1911 and 1913, respectively, in order to develop their own systems.

Brilliant clinical ophthalmic surgeons and outstanding experimentally minded research ophthalmalogists developed during the early years of the twentieth century, particularly in German and Austrian clinics.

Morphine and scopalamine ("twilight sleep") were used in obstetrics in 1902 and barbiturates were commonly given prior to general anesthesia. However, the specialty of anesthesiology was not to develop until between World Wars I and II.

Thoracic surgery was developed to a considerable degree prior to World War I. Artificial pneumothorax treatment for tuberculosis was proposed by Carlo Forlanini of Pavia, in 1882, and was introduced into the United States by Doctor John B. Murphy of Chicago. The first successful resection of the pulmonary apex for tuberculosis was done by Doctor Theodore Tuffier of Paris in 1891 and Sir William McEwen of Glasgow was the first to excise an entire necrotic lung in 1895. Franz Torek of New York did the first successful thoraco-esophagectomy in 1913, Samuel J. Meltzer of New York introduced intratracheal insufflation anesthesia, Morton B. Kirschner of Breslau did the first successful pulmonary embolectomy, Ludwig Rehn of Marburg accomplished the first successful suture of a heart wound, Carl Beck of New York did pioneer work in the surgery of empyema and of the esophagus, Sir Lauder Brunton of London was the first to suggest and to carry out experiments on the surgery for mitral stenosis and Paul L.

Friedrich of Leipzig was the first to do thoracoplasty.

The majority of the present-day medical and surgical specialties had been introduced prior to World War I. Physical medicine and rehabilitation, cardiac surgery, pediatric surgery, oncology and a number of subspecialties emerged later.

Group medical practice was introduced prior to World War I. This system reached its epitome in the development of the Mayo Clinic in Rochester, Minnesota. This clinic was developed from the medical and surgical practices of Doctors W. W. Mayo, W. J. Mayo, and C. H. Mayo and associates. Because of the professional and organizational excellence of this group, it was reorganized as the Mayo Foundation for Medical Education and Research in 1915.

Nobel Prizewinners in medicine and physiology during the twentieth century prior to World War I are listed below.

| *Date* | *Winners* | *Nationality* | *Contributions* |
|---|---|---|---|
| 1901 | Emil von Behring | German | The discoverer of diphtheria and tetanus antitoxin. |
| 1902 | Sir Ronald Ross | British | The discoverer of the transmission of malaria by mosquitoes. |
| 1903 | Neil Finsen | Danish | Pioneer in heliotherapy. |
| 1904 | Ivan Pavlov | Russian | Physiologist who made epochal studies on digestion. |
| 1905 | Robert Koch | German | A founder of modern bacteriology and discoverer of the tubercle bacillus. |
| 1906 | Santiago Ramõn y Cajal | Spanish | Pioneer in the study of the finer anatomy of the nervous system. |
| 1907 | Charles Laveran | French | Discoverer of the malarial parasite. |
| 1908 | Paul Ehrlich | German | Father of modern chemotherapy and hematology. |
| 1909 | Theodor Kocher | Swiss | Surgeon, for his investigations on goitre. |
| 1910 | Albrecht Kossel | German | Physiologist who made outstanding discoveries in the chemistry of the cell and the cell nucleus. |
| 1911 | Allvar Gullstrand | Swedish | Discovered the intracapsular mechanism of accommodation. |
| 1912 | Alexis Carrel | French | Studied extra-vital cultivation and rejuvenation of tissues and the transplantation of organs. |
| 1913 | Charles Richet | French | Physiologist, discoverer of anaphylaxis. |
| 1914 | Robert Barany | Austrian | Otorhino-laryngologist, discoverer of the tests for vestibular function. |

## MEDICINE: WORLD WAR I TO WORLD WAR II

World War I brought to an end the Victorian era and resulted in marked political, economical, social and scientific changes. The war had many causes but actually began over a dispute in the Balkans. Franz Ferdinand, heir to the Hapsburg throne, was assassinated by a southern Slav patriot at Sarajevo in Bosnia in 1914. An ultimatum was issued by the Austrian Government to put an end to agitation by the southern Slavs but this was rejected. The allies of the nations so involved were called upon to support their treaties. The Serbs, therefore, were supported by Russia, France stood by its obligations to Russia and Britain supported France. Germany felt obliged to stand by its ally, Austria, and World War I began. Csarist Russia was the first to suffer total defeat. This led to disorganization and discontent in Russia and thence to revolution in March of 1917. The United States intervened in March of 1917. The Communists seized power in Russia in October of 1917 and took that country out of the war, which finally ended when the German and Austro-Hungarian empires collapsed in 1918.

Territorial settlements were made following World War I on the basis of the principle of national self-determination. Various linguistic groups emerged as sovereign states in eastern Europe.

The great depression of the early 1930's weakened the Weimer Republic and made many Germans receptive to Adolf Hitler and the claims of the Nazi Party. The Nazis obtained control of Germany in 1933 and, in following years, repudiated the various clauses of the treaties that had been made after World War I. Hitler reoccupied the Rhineland with German troops and announced a program of German rearmament in 1936. In the same year, both Germany and Italy tested their weapons in the Spanish Civil War. Hitler then proceeded to occupy those countries which he stated were populated by ethnic Germans outside Germany itself. In March of 1939, the Nazis occupied the Slavic countries of Bohemia and Moravia, thus indicating German aims to subjugate Europe itself. When Poland was invaded by the Germans and then by the Russians, Britain, having guaranteed Poland, declared war on Germany as did France on September 3, 1939. World War II had begun.

After the Bolshevik Revolution on November 7, 1917, the second All-Russian Congress of Soviets opened with a majority which accepted Lenin's leadership. Russia faced a desperate problem of economic reconstruction after World War I. The economy was planned in order to end all free enterprise and private trade, except for the sale of produce that farmers grew on their small household plots. These reforms destroyed the newly rich trading class and the previously successful farmers. The Soviet foreign policy aimed at organizing Communist revolutions throughout the world and the Comintern was especially active in China during this time. The United States reestablished diplomatic relations with the Soviet Union in 1933 and the U.S.S.R. entered the League of Nations in 1934. The Seventh Comintern Congress in 1935 ordered Communist authorities throughout the world to join with antifascist parties in the development of "popular front" organizations. The beginning of World War II saw Russia involved in a nonaggression pact with the Nazis. These events had profound effects upon medical practice and science during this era in all countries.

*World War I was the first war of magnitude in history in which the mortality from battle casualties exceeded that from communicable diseases. The next greatest medical achievement of the war was the control of wound infection.* The death rate from wounds which were treated in the hospital was reduced by one-half in comparison to that from injuries sustained and treated during the Civil War. In addition, every soldier was a potential bacillus carrier because of his exposure to trench warfare. The physical-chemical principle of wound irrigation with a solution of a gas in a liquid (Carrel-Dakin) and later the mechanical principle of debridement and primary suture were thought to have contributed to the improved results in the control of wound infection. Carrel-Dakin irrigation consisted of the use of a solution which set free chlorine gas and was a refinement of previous antiseptic methods.

Maxillofacial surgery, the treatment of gunshot fractures, and roentgenography advanced remarkably during this period. Psychology and neuropsychiatry proved to be valuable in the selection of individuals who were fit for military service and in the study of the syndrome of "shell-shock." (*Shell-shock* of World War I and *combat-fatigue* of World War II were probably the same conditions and stimulated further advances in psychiatry.) Wound shock, gunshot wound of peripheral nerves, communicable diseases, orthopedic surgery, neurological surgery, aviation medicine and poisonings from war-gas were among the many areas of medicine to advance during World War I.

Following the war, a number of notable achievements occurred. The discoveries of electroencephalography, electron microscopy, sulfonamides, insulin and the therapeutic value of liver in pernicious anemia are a few among many remarkable advances.

Insulin was discovered in the laboratory of Professor J. J. R. Macleod in the University of Toronto by Frederick Banting and Charles H. Best in 1922 when these young men were thirty and twenty-three years of age, respectively. The development of insulin revolutionized the treatment of diabetes mellitus.

George Whipple and Robscheit-Robbins pointed out the beneficial effect of raw beef liver upon blood regeneration in severe experimental anemia in 1925. George Minot and William P. Murphy of Boston applied this to a patient suffering from pernicious anemia and found that the anemia disappeared and that the red blood count returned to normal, thus establishing the therapeutic value of liver in pernicious anemia.

Sulfonamides were discovered by Gerhard Domagk, German bacteriologist, in 1935. Although he was awarded the Nobel Prize in medicine in 1939 for his remarkable work, Adolf Hitler and his regime would not allow him to accept this. Domagk also found that Prontosil, sulfanilamide-dyestuff, protected mice against fatal doses of hemolytic staphylococci. Sulfanilamides were soon employed for infection in patients and excellent results were obtained. Whitby introduced sulfapyridine, a derivative of sulfanilamide, for the treatment of pneumococcal infections in 1938. This reduced the current mortality of pneumonia by one third. Perrin-Long and Richard Robblin introduced sulfathiazole and sulfadiazine, respectively, in 1940. The latter was found to be a remarkable value in the treatment of various forms of meningitis. Thus, antibiotics and chemotherapy were advanced.

Electroencephalography was developed by Doctor Hans Berger, a German physician, in 1929. This technique has proven to be as important in the diagnosis of cerebral disease as the electrocardiograph has been in the diagnosis of heart disease. It has led to electrocorticography (the recording from the exposed cerebral cortex), depth electrode studies (recording from subcortical areas of the brain) and microelectrode studies (recording from single cells in the nervous system).

The first electron microscope was constructed by Knoll and Ruska in 1931 in Germany. This instrument has been applied to medical science only since the end of World War II and is still in its infancy.

It has now been perfected to produce more than 200,000 magnifications and offers great promise for better understanding of the ultrastructure and functioning of tissues and cells.

Nobel Prizewinners in medicine and physiology are illustrative of the genius and productivity of this inter-war period. They are listed as follows:

| *Date* | *Winners* | *Nationality* | *Contributions* |
|---|---|---|---|
| 1919 | Jules Bordet | Belgian | Discoverer of complement fixation and pioneer student of bacterial hemolysins and bacteriolysis. |
| 1920 | August Krogh | Danish | Made important discoveries on the anatomy and physiology of the capillaries. |
| 1922 | Otto Meyerhof | German | Pioneer in the study of tissue respiration, for his research on the oxidation and utilization of lactic acid in muscles. |
| 1922 | A. V. Hill | English | For studies on the physiology of muscular contraction. |
| 1923 | Frederick G. Banting | Canadian | Discoverers of insulin. |
| | J. J. R. Macleod | Canadian | |
| 1924 | Willem Einthoven | Dutch | Inventor of the electrocardiograph. |
| 1926 | Johannes Fibiger | Danish | Pathologist, made important studies on cancer. |
| 1927 | Julius Wagner von Jauregg | Austrian | Discoverer of fever therapy for general paresis. |
| 1928 | Charles Nicolle | French | Discovered the transmission of typhus fever by lice. |
| 1929 | Frederick Gowland Hopkins | English | Pioneers in the study of avitaminosis. |
| | Christian Eijkman | Dutch | |
| 1930 | Karl Landsteiner | American | Demonstrated different groups of red blood cells. |
| 1931 | Otto H. Warburg | German | Discovering that enzymes aid in respiration by tissues. |
| 1932 | Edgar D. Adrian | English | Carried out fundamental investigations on the physiology of the nervous system. |
| | Sir Charles S. Sherrington | English | |
| 1933 | Thomas Hunt Morgan | American | Biologist, for his work on genetics and experimental embryology. |
| 1934 | George R. Minot | American | Discovered the therapeutic value of liver in pernicious anemia. |
| | William P. Murphy | American | |
| | George H. Whipple | American | |
| 1935 | Hans Spemann | German | In recognition of his investigations on embryonic evolution, particularly on the causes of organ development. |
| 1936 | Sir Henry H. Dale | British | For their discoveries on the chemical transmission of nerve impulses. |
| | Otto Loewi | Austrian | |
| 1937 | Albert Szent-Gyorgyi von Nagyrapolt | Hungarian | Isolated vitamin C (ascorbic acid) and vitamin P. |
| 1938 | Corneille Heymans | Belgian | Pharmacologist and physiologist, whose work on the functions of the carotid sinus was noteworthy. |

## WORLD WAR II TO THE PRESENT

The Germans under Hitler, during the summer of 1940, controlled the European continent west of Russia and turned to attack Great Britain which was at that time the only power at war with them. After losing the Battle of Britain in the air Hitler invaded Russia in June, 1941.

World War II weakened the British, French and Dutch colonial regimes in Southeast Asia and it is generally conceded that it was American resistance to Japanese plans for the area that brought the Japanese into war with the United States. The bombing of Pearl Harbor on December 7, 1941, by Japan and the invasion of the Philippine Islands, then a possession of the United States, brought the Americans into war with Japan and it's allies, Germany and Italy. The war in Europe ended on

April 30, 1945 and that in the Pacific on August 6, 1945.

The number of civilian deaths, though unknown, probably exceeded the number of military fatalities for the first time in many generations in conflicts of civilized peoples, not only because of the bombings, but because of the policies of deliberate extermination of the Jews and others on the part of the Nazis. The war left the United States and the Soviet Union as the two strongest military and industrial powers. Each feared (and still does) the spread of the influence of the other in the world and both are armed with atomic and thermonuclear weapons. Smaller emerging nations, their conflicts, and the continuing ideological differences among the powers have resulted in the Korean, Vietnamese and the Middle East Wars. These conflicts have occurred in a period of twenty years after World War II, in spite of the United Nations Organization, which was founded at the end of World War II in an attempt to settle international differences by means of diplomacy.

The Soviet Communist Party has recently celebrated the fiftieth anniversary of the Bolshevik Revolution of November 7, 1917 and restated that "peaceful coexistence" remains the basis of its international relations and that the main struggle in the world of today was the ideological fight between the Communist and the Capitalist. This thesis, the same as that of Marx, is:

> There is not and there can not be any neutralism in the struggle against the bourgeois ideology and anti-Communism. This is a class struggle, a struggle for man, for the triumph of freedom and the progress of humanity.

It is obvious that this conflict has complex origins, no easy solutions and considerable selective imperception by all concerned. In spite of international problems, medicine has accelerated remarkably in its advance since World War II.

The population crisis, factors of health and wealth, the major killing and crippling diseases, advances in nursing and patterns in medical progress are among significant elements of medicine of the twentieth century. Each, of course, is based upon the experience of previous generations.

## POPULATION CRISIS

The rate of growth of the human race is one-hundred and eighty-nine thousand daily. This means that the pace of world population growth has more than doubled since 1945 and that the total population of the world now is estimated at 3.4 billion people.

Modern medicine and sanitation have cut death rates dramatically even though birth rates remain unchanged in much of the world. The rate of increase is now at least seven times what it was two centuries ago. It will take just another thirty-five years to reach more than seven billion people (approximately twice the present population).

Unfortunately, two-thirds of the people are underfed or undernourished, and economic as well as social progress is slow in comparison to the rate of increase in population. We may expect our rapid increase in numbers to burden rather than to accelerate our economy, because industrial productivity from the standpoint of living determines purchasing power rather than the number of people. Food production distribution and birth control measures may develop sufficiently to alleviate the situation somewhat. The problems as well as the solutions are extremely complex and medicine will be intimately involved with them for years to come.

## HEALTH AND WEALTH

It is estimated that illness results in a loss of income of approximately 2.4 billion dollars annually and that private expenditures for health and medical services amount to approximately twenty-seven billion dollars annually—or a total of almost thirty billion dollars each year in the United States. The United States Public Health Service will spend 2.6 billion dollars in 1968 to find new treatments and cures for cancer, cardiovascular diseases, mental illnesses, arthritis and metabolic diseases, neurological and blinding eye diseases, allergic and infectious diseases and dental disorders. Major voluntary health agencies will spend approximately forty-million dollars for similar purposes. Departments of the Federal Government other than the Public Health Service spend over four-hundred million dollars annually on medical and "health related" research.

According to the *Statistical Abstract of the United States, 1965*, from the United States Department of Commerce, Bureau of Census, personal consumption expenditure by type of product (1963) was as follows:

| | |
|---|---|
| Food, beverages and tobacco | $ 95,200,000,000 |
| Household operations | 52,400,000,000 |
| Housing | 48,900,000,000 |
| Transportation | 47,200,000,000 |
| Clothing, accessories and jewelry | 37,100,000,000 |
| *Medical care and death expenses* | 25,400,000,000 |
| Personal business | 24,900,000,000 |
| Recreation | 22,700,000,000 |
| Personal care (other than medical) | 6,500,000,000 |
| Private education and research | 5,700,000,000 |
| Religious and welfare activities | 5,400,000,000 |
| Foreign travel and remittances | 3,500,000,000 |
| *Total Personal Consumption Expenditures, 1963* | $375,000,000,000 |

More persons are employed today by hospitals than by the automobile industry. Needed expansion for hospitals is of vital importance for the construction industry which is basic in the United States economy and hospital construction during the current year will approximate two billion dollars. Long-term construction of needed facilities will require an estimated outlay of twenty-three billion dollars. During the period from 1955 to 1960, the cost of hospitalization has increased about four times in comparison to physicians' fees, eight times as much as drugs and prescriptions and nearly four times as much as the increase in the general consumers' goods price index. This is because hospitals have been burdened by equipment costs, rapidly increasing labor costs and the declining ability of personal philanthropy to bridge the gap between income and expenses. Labor costs amount to two thirds of the expenses of hospitalization. Approximately 75 percent of the population is covered by prepaid medical insurance in the United States. Medicare for the aged under the Social Security Administration and medical plans for all citizens are being formulated. Medicine is totally socialized in Russia and is becoming more so in the United States. The National Health Service, which was instituted in 1948, in Great Britain, has met some of the basic needs of the population. New adjustments along medical lines will continually be necessary because of the changing social and medical needs in the world.

The most costly disease known to mankind on a worldwide basis is malaria. It still affects one-hundred and forty countries and territories. The World Health Organization has an estimated cost of 1.7 billion dollars in order to accomplish the control of this disease. Money, therefore, plays a major role in controlling or eradicating the major killing and crippling diseases of our time.

## MAJOR KILLING AND CRIPPLING DISEASES

Malaria, pneumonia, tuberculosis, gastritis (including duodenitis, enteritis, colitis) and other infectious and parasitic diseases represent those which cause the greatest death toll in underdeveloped countries. The knowledge to control or prevent these diseases is known but has not been applied widely or effectively.

Leading causes of death in the western world are about the same in all countries and are as follows:

1. Heart diseases (heart attack)—basic cause: arteriosclerosis;
2. Cancer, and
3. Vascular lesions (stroke)—basic cause: arteriosclerosis.

The leading killers in the United States in 1965 were as follows:

| | |
|---|---|
| 1. Cardiovascular-renal diseases: | |
| Heart diseases | 709,010 |
| "Strokes" | 203,330 |
| Hypertension | 66,810 |
| 2. Cancer and other malignant tumors | 296,320 |
| 3. Accidents | 106,900 |
| 4. Pneumonia, except pneumonia of newborn, influenza (2,150 deaths) | 61,460 |
| 5. Certain diseases of early infancy (birth injuries, postnatal asphyxia, atelectasis, infections of newborns) | 55,060 |
| 6. Diabetes mellitus | 33,170 |
| 7. Broncho-pulmonary diseases | 32,670 |
| 8. Cirrhosis of the liver | 24,250 |
| 9. Suicide | 22,560 |
| 10. Congenital malformations | 19,730 |

Total estimated deaths in 1965 were 1,825,000. There were 1,150 maternal deaths and 93,200 infant deaths (under one year of age) with 71 percent of these dying during the first twenty-eight days.

Disabling and crippling conditions have been reported to involve approximately 45 percent of the civilian, noninstitutionalized population of the United States according to a recently published National Health Survey. The estimated number of people so afflicted is tabulated as follows:

| | | |
|---|---|---|
| 1. Mental and emotional disorders | | 19,000,000 |
| 2. Diseases of heart and circulation, including Cerebrovascular diseases (mainly due to arteriosclerosis) | | 16,421,000 |
| 3. Arthritis and rheumatic diseases | | 13,000,000 |
| 4. Neurological disorders | | 10,000,000 |
| Epilepsy | 1,800,000 | |
| Cerebral palsy | 550,000 | |
| Multiple sclerosis and Demyelinating diseases | 500,000 | |
| Parkinson's disease | 500,000 | |
| Muscular dystrophy | 200,000 | |
| 5. Hearing impairments | | 6,231,000 |
| 6. Mentally retarded | | 5,400,000 |
| 7. Visual impairments | | 3,500,000 |
| Legally Blind—416,400 | | |
| 12,000,000 children need eye care | | |
| 8. Diabetes mellitus | | 1,500,000 |
| 9. Cancer (estimated under treatment now) | | 870,000 |

Triumphs over infection have greatly prolonged life and health in the western world. A sharp rise in diseases of the heart may reflect the increased speed and stress of living, in that they ranked fourth in 1900 but are today by far the leading cause of death. Of interest is that accidental deaths occur most commonly between the ages of one and twenty-four, next between twenty-five and forty-four and with least frequency after the age of forty-five. The death rate from cancer and other malignant neoplasms at the present time is more than double what it was in 1900 and now accounts for one of every six deaths. Although diseases of the early infancy have declined, the rate of congenital malformations has persisted.

Life expectancy at the time of birth in underdeveloped countries ranges from around thirty years for both men and women but is as high as seventy for men and seventy-five for women in countries that are more highly developed.

## ADVANCES IN NURSING

Beginning with the first mother down to the present day, women have protected children, have cared for the elderly and sick members of the family and have also offered their services to neighbors during illness.

Nursing was nurtured in the early Christian period. One of the earliest groups of women workers were the Deaconesses who were particularly concerned with visiting and nursing the sick and in distributing alms. A friend of St. Paul, Phoebe was the first Deaconess and, thus, the first visiting nurse. The Order of Deaconesses later adopted a distinctive garb, attained a position of some importance for many years, but gradually disappeared. Some noble Roman matrons, after conversion to Christianity, founded hospitals and convents and also distinguished themselves in the field of nursing.

During the early Middle Ages, the twin sister of St. Benedict, St. Scholastica, founded an order for women based on the Benedictine Rule near Monte Cassino. She held the office of Abbess and, along with other famous women of the Benedictine Order, contributed to the field of nursing. The Hótel Dieu in Lyons, established in 1542, was a famous medieval hospital in which nursing was carried out by repentent women, by widows called sisters (not a religious group) and by male nurses called brothers. The oldest nursing Order of Sisters in existence was founded by the Augustinian Sisters who formed a religious order from what originally had been the nursing staff of the Hótel Dieu in Paris which was founded in 1650.

The formation of military nursing orders during the Crusades has been discussed previously. In addition, a sisterhood of nurses was formed to staff the hospitals and to free Hospitallers for nursing on the battle front and for fighting. These nurses were the Sisters of the Order of St. John of Jerusalem. Secular nursing orders were also founded during the eleventh and twelfth centuries.

The "dark period" of nursing extended from about 1600 until the middle of the nineteenth century, largely because the Reformation had eliminated the presence of religious orders in hundreds of hospitals.

The Irish Sisters of Charity were founded in 1815, by Mother Mary Aikenhead who had been trained in England. This order did social work, visiting and hospital nursing. Hospitals were then established in Dublin and elsewhere. They went to Australia in 1857 and founded hospital work there. The Sisters of Mercy were founded near Dublin in 1828 by Mother Catherine McAuley, the first women under religious auspices to be permitted, since the days of the Reformation, to enter the public hospitals of the United Kingdom and care for the sick. The Sisters of Mercy nursed the wounded on the battlefields of the Crimean War, the soldiers of the Union and Confederate Armies in the Civil War, and in the Spanish-American War. The Army, Navy and Red Cross nursing services have continued this work and the Sisters serve their countries now in time of war by planning for disaster and rendering nursing care to the civilian population. The Sisters of Mercy are presently the largest English-speaking religious nursing order and second numerically to the Daughters of Charity.

Daughters of Charity were founded in 1633 by St. Vincent de Paul and became a secular nursing order of high character. A systematic educational program was set up consisting of experiences in the hospital, visiting in homes and caring for the sick there. The Daughters of Charity now comprise the largest religious nursing community in the world and are largely French-speaking.

The Protestant Sisters of Charity were established by Elizabeth Fry in England about 1840. This group was given training but their practical experience was merely by observing patients in London hospitals. Other sisterhoods were formed during this period and some of these nurses were chosen by Florence Nightingale for her work in the Crimean War. These orders were the immediate forerunners of modern schools of nursing.

Florence Nightingale is generally considered to be the founder of modern nursing. She was born on May 12, 1820 in Florence, Italy and received a wide education. Even as a youngster, she indicated a desire to nurse the sick. Nursing was not considered to be a proper career for young women of her station, but she persisted in her goal, visited and studied hospitals in France, Germany, Belgium and Italy, having already seen those in Great Britain, and in 1851, enrolled for three months of training. She also worked with the Sisters of Charity in Paris and her first position was as superintendent of the Establishment for Gentle Women during Illness. She was then requested to assume the new post of Superintendent of Nurses at Kings College Hospital in London. Just before doing so, she was called to go to the Crimea. Within a period of one week she had chosen her nurses, thirty-eight in all, and they were assigned to the Base Hospital at Scutari where they had charge of 1,500 patients. She transformed the hospital into an efficiently-managed institution and her compassion during her nightly rounds gave her the title of "The Lady of the Lamp." The Irish Sisters of Mercy had also sent fifteen sisters to the Crimea at about the same time as Miss Nightingale. They worked nearby and also distinguished themselves. These successes in nursing led to gradual acceptance of nursing as a profession, due to the demonstrated ability and devotion of these women. During the 1870's, the first schools of nursing in the United States were founded, and there was an increase in the number of schools developed in Great Britain and elsewhere. Nursing has followed step-by-step with advances in medicine during this century, including the development of textbooks by nurses, specialties and ever-expanding curricula and opportunities. There is a growing trend among nursing associations to favor education as provided by universities rather than by hospitals. The present position of the American Medical Association is to support all forms of nursing education, including a strong endorsement of diploma or hospital-based schools of nursing.

The place of the future professional nurse in her field of nursing and in our larger society has been expressed by the National Nursing Council as follows:

> It is the opinion of this group that in the latter half of the twentieth century, the professional nurse will be the one who recognizes and understands the fundamental (health) needs of a person, sick or well, and who knows how these needs can best be met. She will possess a body of scientific nursing knowledge which is based upon and keeps pace with general scientific advancement and she will be able to apply this knowledge in meeting the nursing needs of a person and a community. She must possess that kind of discriminative judgment which will enable her to recognize those activities which fall within the area of professional nursing and those activities which have been identified with the fields of other professional or nonprofessional groups.
>
> She must be able to exert leadership in at least four different ways; (1) in making her unique contribution to the preventive and remedial aspects of illness; (2) improving those nursing skills already in existence and developing new nursing skills; (3) in teaching and supervising other nurses and auxiliary workers and (4) in cooperating with other professions in planning for positive health on community, state, national and international levels.

## PATTERNS OF MEDICAL PROGRESS

The impact of the wars of the twentieth century have not made mankind happier, wiser or morally better and so, if medicine is not measured according to these values, considerable progress has been made. Certainly prevention, control and cure of disease are more effective and widespread than at any time before in history. As in the past, physicians still must function within the cultural environment in which they live. Some recent trends in a few countries will illustrate this fact.

### U.S.S.R.

Medical service in the Soviet Union is directed by the Ministry of Health in Moscow. Each of the fifteen Soviet Socialist Republics has its own ministry also. There are two organizations which are responsible for medical education. The majority of medical training is under the aegis of the Ministry of Health, but there are six medical faculties at universities under the Ministry of Higher Education. There are some 130 establishments making up a network of research institutes and laboratories as well as "construction bureaus," the latter having to do with the production of apparatus and drugs. Basic medical training takes six years and is available in eighty-six establishments in the U.S.S.R. There are also twenty-three centers where qualified doctors may train for higher qualifications. In addition, there are more than 300 specialist centers in research institutes. For example, there are institutes for the study of cancer, virology, tuberculosis, obstetrics and gynecology, lung diseases, cardiology, neurology and neurosurgery, gastroenterology, and for work on plastic materials and medicine, to name a few. Soviet surgeons have successfully transplanted organs. Of interest is the fact that the present Minister of Health, Doctor Boris V. Petrovski was awarded the Lenin Prize for his work on kidney transplantation. He performed the first such operation in the U.S.S.R. early in 1965 before he became Minister and continues to combine the roles of medical administrator and practicing surgeon. There are ninety centers in the Soviet Union equipped with artificial kidney machines. The prototype of the heart-lung machines now used in Soviet hospitals was developed in the 30's and open-heart surgery is actively practiced. Soviet medical sciences are continuing to score considerable success in different lines of research and a large number of the physicians, surgeons and medical scientists are women.

### Poland

The Ministry of Health controls fourteen scientific institutes and ten academies, or schools of medicine. In addition, there are ten research centers which draw annual or long-term plans for research in the indicated problem areas. Several annual awards are given each year to those whose work is considered most valuable by the state committee. The top award in 1966 went to a surgeon who had specialized in a low temperature surgical instrument to remove cataracts. The use of his cryoextractor to remove the lens had been successfully employed on more than 2,000 patients. Another function of the Scientific Board of the Ministry of Health is to collect information on developments in medicine in other countries.

### Bulgaria

Medical development is also directed in a similar fashion. More than 1,500 medical scientific workers are now occupied in research work in Bulgaria.

### Italy

Most of the hospitals of Italy were founded and operated on the initiative of religious, community or private groups. At present, the Ministry of Health has proposed reorganization of the hospitals under a national scheme but this is still controversial. The present national medical social security plan has led to widespread "paperwork strikes" by Italian physicians and the Italian medical community is in a ferment of modernization.

### Spain

The leading causes of death in Spain are similar to those in other western countries. Cardiovascular disease is the leading killer, followed by cancer. Industrial and traffic accidents are the third most frequent cause of death. Spanish hospitals are being modernized and advanced techniques have been introduced in treatment of vascular, respiratory, and nervous systems, as well as other specialties. The introduction of the Sabine vaccine has been credited with bringing about a 95 percent drop in poliomyelitis. Tuberculosis control is still a problem, although the mortality rate has declined.

### Sweden

The Swedish medical associations are presently recommending reorganization in the present structure of providing care to the healthy and to the sick. The National Swedish Welfare Board now administers medical care for all who are healthy and the National Board of Health is in charge of those who are ill. The medical associations have recommended that these two agencies combine or at least streamline into a central administration, but the means for accomplishing this have not been achieved as yet.

The Northern Federation of Medical Teachers includes representatives from Denmark, Finland, Iceland, Norway and Sweden and is presently working out a plan to shorten the course leading to a medical degree to five and one-half years. The Karolinska Institute continues its contributions to world medicine and science and to select the Nobel Prizewinners in medicine and physiology. Other Scandinavian institutions and individuals are providing outstanding work.

### Switzerland

The quality of Swiss medicine and surgery remains high by international standards. Parliament has been requested by the Swiss Academy of Medical Sciences and all medical facilties to form a national health research fund because of inadequate support by the government and other agencies for research in the past. The specialty of physical medicine and rehabilitation has developed widely in Switzerland in recent years. Because of a relatively small population, the various universities in Switzerland have specialized, have concentrated patients and facilities and established reputations in certain aspects of medicine.

### Great Britain

The National Health Service was instituted in 1948, along with other social reforms in response to the will of the electorate. Since then, particularly because of economic problems, there has been a lag in construction of new hospitals and considerable physical decay of existing hospitals. The physicians have adjusted to the lowered income, but not without considerable alarm about the future of the National Health Service. A rather continuous drift of young doctors to other countries has resulted in vacancies in the hospitals being filled with thousands of doctors from Africa, India, the West Indies and Pakistan. The government is attempting to increase the pay for doctors and the Ministry of Health has announced a new hospital building plan. There has been an increase in small private hospitals in order to meet the needs of the increasing number of people who now choose to pay for hospital care outside of the National Health Service.

### Canada

Between 1945 and 1955, the development of medical schools was slow because of relatively poor support for medical research. Since 1955, the government has found it necessary to more adequately support medical education in order to maintain quality, to expand facilities and to do creative work. The new Canadian medical system provides a program for hospital insurance in which hospital care for any resident is paid for jointly by the provincial and federal governments. Every kind of medical practice is found in Canada because of its varied geography and regional differences and these elements have prevented both the profession and the politicians from making indiscriminate generalizations on an overall plan. There has been a tremendous increase in hospital building in Canada since 1950 and a special Health Resouces Fund for the expansion and equipping of these teaching hospitals and research institutions indicates that this development is likely to continue. Approximately 30 percent of the younger Canadian physicians were lured south of the border during the past year. This results in the problem of training and keeping personnel, even though well-equipped hospital facilities are available in most communities.

## Argentina

Students begin their clinical training and then are sent to different city hospitals where they remain at the same hospital for a period of three years. A modified teaching system in the schools has been established because of the shortage of teachers after a basic period of instruction in the medical schools themselves. Centers for respiratory rehabilitation, for chronic renal failure, for cardiological and other specialties have been developed.

## Brazil

Schistosomiasis and tetanus have been very common and serious problems in Brazil but medications and immunization therapy have resulted in a marked reduction in the incidence of these conditions. Consistent success in renal homotransplantation procedures by a unit in the faculty of medicine at the University of São Paulo is an indication of the achievement possible in this region.

## El Salvador

The main medical problems in El Salvador are communicable disease, malnutrition, inadequate sanitation and acts of violence. More than half of the population is under twenty years of age and criminal abortion has become one of the most important social problems. The government has steadily increased its annual public health budget.

## Mexico

Approximately 25 percent of the national budget is now allocated to the improvement of health services and social security in Mexico. Vigorous measures against communicable diseases are proving to be very effective. Tuberculosis, however, is still among the first ten causes of death and infectious diseases are responsible for 5.6 percent of hospital admissions (1966). Infant mortality has dropped and life expectancy in Mexico is now sixty-six years, which is a gain of about seven years over the figure of four years previously. Although 48 percent of the 1,200 beds in Mexico are considered to be private, they average only about 18 percent of the total number of beds. Three systems of medical care as well as disability and retirement pension are provided by the Mexican Social Security Institute and the Government Workers' Social Services and Security Institute. Approximately thirty-one million people are cared for directly by the government or by private medical practitioners and not by social security. The National Medical Center has over 2,000 beds and a number of specialty institutes.

## United States

Perhaps the outstanding pattern of medical change in the United States during the past two decades has been the skyrocketing of support for medical care and education by the Public Health Service. There has been a corresponding reduction in private and corporate philanthropy which has been attributed to taxation and some loss of incentive for donors in this field. Universities, medical schools and hospitals, as well as research institutes, have been directly affected by these changes in the sources of support. The total appropriation for the Public Health Service—including the National Institutes of Health—for fiscal 1968 was 2.6 billion dollars. The National Library of Medicine is now the largest in the world. It started as a library of the Surgeon General and in due time became the Army Medical Library. It was transferred from the Department of Defense to the Department of Health, Education and Welfare in 1956 and has since been called the National Library of Medicine. This library houses more than one million volumes, serves libraries elsewhere and individual physicians upon request.

Continuous monitoring of the electrocardiogram, pulse and blood pressure have become standard in coronary care units. Cardiac arrest teams have been developed so that the defibrillators, internal and external pacemakers and respiratory equipment are commonplace in major hospitals. Heart surgery has continued to develop as one of the most exciting fields of medicine. Inhalation therapy units have also been developed and have proved their worth to patients. The problems of disease of pulmonary insufficiency persist. Although thoracic surgery has advanced so that cancer of the lung can be successfully treated in some cases, the frequency of this condition continues to increase alarmingly. Some headway is being made in the continuing effort to protect human beings immunologically against the vast army of viruses and bacteria. Some progress toward a better understanding of the immune mechanisms underlying the allergic states has developed. The remarkable advances in radiology, including image amplifiers, the use of isotopes, scanning techniques and echoencephalography, as well as television monitors and cineradiography have emanated from a number of centers in the United States and abroad and are now commonplace in major medical centers. It is not possible to do justice to the remarkable challenges in each of the fields of medicine and nursing in the space of this chapter.

Specialization has become so interesting * and attractive to the medical profession in recent years and the knowledge explosion so immense, that the American Medical Association appointed a Citizens' Commission on Graduate Medical Education. Their report was published on August 1, 1966. An American Board of Primary Medicine (General Practice) has been recommended as well as specialty training in general practice, in order to revive and encourage the important work of the family physician. Other recommendations included the dropping of the traditional internship, the reorganization of various types of residency training programs and the creation of the new Commission on Graduate Medical Education. This commission would have the authority to plan, coordinate and to periodically review standards for graduate medical education and the procedures for reviewing and improving the institutions in which that education is offered. Some of these recommendations have already been activated, but others are controversial and will undoubtedly be modified before acceptance in the future.

The work of the Nobel Prizewinners since 1939 attests to the quality, quantity and international flavor of medicine. They are listed as follows:

* Eighty-four percent of all physicians that work in private practice reported themselves to be general practitioners in 1931 and only 37 percent reported similarly in 1965.

| Date | Winners | Nationality | Contributions |
|---|---|---|---|
| 1939 | Gerhard Domagk | German | Bacteriologist, discovered the therapeutic value of sulphanilamides. |
| 1943 | Henrik Dam | Danish | For discovering and synthesizing vitamin K. |
| | Edward A. Doisy | American | |
| 1944 | Joseph Erlanger | Americans | Physiologists, for their work on action current of nerves. |
| | Herbert Gasser | | |
| 1945 | Sir Alexander Fleming | British | Bacteriologists, discovered penicillin. |
| | Sir Howard W. Florey | British | |
| | Ernest B. Chain | British | |
| 1946 | Herman Joseph Müller | American | Biologist, produced mutations by the employment of x-rays. |
| 1947 | Carl F. and | American | For their discovery of the process in the catalytic metabolism of glycogen. |
| | Gerty Cori | | |
| | Bernardo Houssay | Argentinian | Physiologist, for his work on role of the anterior pituitary hormone in the distribution of glycogen in the body and control of diabetes. |
| 1948 | Paul Mueller | Swiss | Discovered that DDT was an effective insecticide. |
| 1949 | Walter F. Hess | Swiss | For his studies on the reaction of animals to electric shock. |
| | Antonio E. Moniz | Portuguese | Devised and perfected prefrontal lobotomy. |
| 1950 | Philip S. Hench | American | For their work on pituitary adreno-cortico-tropic hormone (ACTH) and cortisone (Compound E). |
| | Edward C. Kendall | American | |
| | Tadeus Reichstein | Swiss | |
| 1951 | Max Theiler | American | For developing the yellow fever vaccine known as 17-D. |
| 1952 | Selman A. Waksman | American | Discovery of streptomycin. |
| 1953 | Fritz Albert Lipmann | American | For their discoveries in biosynthesis and metabolism. |
| | Hans Adolph Krebs | British | |
| 1954 | John F. Enders | American | For discovering a simple method of growing polio virus in test tubes. |
| | Thomas H. Weller | American | |
| | Frederick C. Robbins | American | |
| 1955 | Hugo Theorell | Swedish | For his discoveries on the nature and action of oxidation enzymes. |
| 1956 | Andre F. Cournand | American | For using a catheter to chart the interior of the heart. |
| | Dickinson W. Richards, Jr. | American | |
| | Werner Forssmann | German | |
| 1957 | Daniel Bovet | Italian | For discovering antihistamines. |
| 1958 | George Wells Beadle | American | For their pioneering work in biochemical genetics. |
| | Edward Lawrie Tatum | American | |
| | Joshua Lederberg | American | For his studies of genetics in bacteria. |
| 1959 | Severo Ochoa | American | For discovering a way to produce nucleic acid by artificial means. |
| | Arthur Kornberg | American | |
| 1960 | Sir Frank M. Burnet | Australian | For research in transplanting human organs. |
| | Peter B. Medawar | British | |
| 1961 | George von Bekesy | American | Discoveries concerning physical mechanism of stimulation within cochlea. |
| 1962 | Francis H. C. Crick | British | Discovery of molecular structure of DNA, substance which controls heredity. |
| | James D. Watson | American | |
| | Maurice H. F. Wilkins | British | |
| 1963 | Alan Lloyd Hodgkin | British | Mathematical analysis of discharge-recovery cycle of nerve cells transmitting nerve impulses. |
| | Andrew F. Huxley | British | |
| | Sir John C. Eccles | Australian | Explanation of travel of nerve impulses across junction between nerve cells. |
| 1964 | Conrad E. Block | American | Research into the relationship between heart disease and cholesterol. |
| | Feodor Lynen | German | |
| 1965 | Francois Jacob | French | Discovery of regulatory activities inside body cells that contribute to the "genetic control of enzymes and virus synthesis." |
| | Andre Lwoff | French | |
| | Jacques Monad | French | |
| 1966 | Peyton Rous | American | Discovery of viral etiology of certain cancers. |
| | Charles Huggins | American | Studies on genital cancer. |
| 1967 | Ragnar Granit | Swedish | Research into the primary chemical and physiological visual processes in the eye. |
| | Holdan K. Hartline | American | |
| | George Wald | American | |

## CONCLUSION

It will be the work of the remainder of the twentieth century and of centuries to come to reduce the major causes of death and crippling and to continue to improve the quality and quantity of medical services, teaching and research for the benefit of society. These objectives can be accomplished if civilization avoids destroying itself, if the political, religious and economic conditions permit, if the minds of men and women are properly motivated and if adequate financial support is provided. The torch in this marathon of life is now yours. The opportunities and challenges are equally great.

*For books are not absolutely dead things, but do contain a potency of life in them to be as active as that soul was whose progency they are; nay, they do preserve as in a vial the purest efficacy and extraction of that living intellect that bred them.*—John Milton

# Recommended Reading List

The following books and periodicals are listed for the purpose of introducing the student to some of the available literature in the field of medical history. Each of these publications will suggest further study.

I *Journals*

1. *Bulletin of the History of Medicine,* Temkin, O. (Ed.): organ of the Amer. Assoc. for the Hist. of Med. and of the Johns Hopkins Institute of the History of Medicine, The Johns Hopkins Press, Baltimore.
2. *Journal of the History of Medicine and Allied Sciences,* Stevenson, L. G. (Ed.): published quarterly from the Department Hist., Science and Medicine, Yale University, New Haven, Connecticut.
3. *M D Medical Newsmagazine,* Martí-Ibáñez, F. (Pres.): M D Publications, New York.
4. Temkin, O.: An essay on the usefulness of medical history for medicine. *Bull Hist Med, 19*:9–47, 1946.

II *General Reference Texts on Medical History*

1. Ackerknecht, E. H.: *A Short History of Medicine.* New York, Ronald, 1955.
2. Bettman, Otto L.: *Pictorial History of Medicine,* Springfield, Ill., Thomas, 1956.
3. Castiglioni, A.: *A History of Medicine,* trans. by Alfred Krumbhaar. Knopf. New York, 1947.
4. Garrison, Fielding H.: *An Introduction to the History of Medicine,* 4th Edit. Philadelphia and London, Saunders, 1949.
5. Gibson, W. C.: *Young Endeavor.* Springfield, Ill., Thomas, 1958.
6. Guthrie, Douglas: *A History of Medicine.* London and New York, Nelson, 1945.
7. Major, Ralph H.: *A History of Medicine,* (2 vols.). Springfield, Ill., Thomas, 1954.
8. Morton, Leslie T.: *Garrison and Morton's Medical Bibliography,* (2nd Ed.). Argosy Bookstore, 114 East 59th Street, New York, 1954.
9. Sigerist, H. E.: *Medicine and Human Welfare.* New Haven, Connecticut, Yale, 1941.

10. Walker, K.: *The Story of Medicine.* New York, Oxford U. P., 1955.

III *Specialty Reference Texts on Medical History*

1. Ackerknecht, Edwin H.: *A Short History of Psychiatry.* New York and London, Hafner, 1959.
2. Arrington, George E.: *A History of Ophthalmology; MD Monographs on Medical History.* New York, MD Pub., 1959.
3. Cianfrani, Theodore: *A Short History of Obstetrics and Gynecology,* Springfield, Ill., Thomas, 1960.
4. Franklin, Kenneth J.: *A Short History of Physiology,* New York, Staples Press, 1949.
5. Haymaker, Webb: *The Founders of Neurology.* Springfield, Ill., Thomas, 1953.
6. Horrax, Gilbert: *Neurosurgery—An Historical Sketch.* Springfield, Ill., Thomas, 1952.
7. Hughes, Arthur: *A History of Cytology.* New York, Abelard, 1959.
8. Hurwitz, A., and Degenshein, G. A.: *Milestones in Modern Surgery.* New York, Hoeber Medical Div., 1958.
9. Keys, Thomas E.: *The History of Surgical Anaesthesia.* New York, Schuman's, 1945.
10. Major, Ralph H.: *Classic Descriptions of Disease.* Springfield, Ill., Thomas, 1948.
11. Meade, Richard H.: *A History of Thoracic Surgery.* Springfield, Ill., Thomas, 1961.
12. Orr, H. W.: *On the Contributions of Hugh Owen Thomas, Sir Robert Jones, and John Ridlon in Modern Orthopedic Surgery.* Springfield, Ill., Thomas, 1960.
13. Sacks, Ernest: *The History and Development of Neurological Surgery.* New York, Hoeber Medical Div., 1952.
14. Walker, A. E.: *A History of Neurological Surgery.* Baltimore, Williams and Wilkins, 1951.
15. Wilkins, Robert H.: *Neurosurgical Classics.* New York, Johnson Reprint, 1965.

IV *Reference Texts on Related Subjects*

1. Bryson, L.: *An Outline of Man's Knowledge of the Modern World.* New York, McGraw, 1960.
2. Field Enterprises Educational Corporation Publishers: *The World Book Encyclopedia* and *The Annual Supplements,* Chicago, 1967.
3. Langer, W. L.: *An Encyclopedia of World History.* Boston, Houghton, 1948.
4. Palmer, R. R.: *Rand-McNally Atlas of World History.* New York, Rand McNally, 1957.
5. Wiener, P. P., and Noland, A.: *Roots of Scientific Thought.* New York, Basic Books, 1957.

V *Primitive and Archaic Medicine*

1. Breasted, James Henry: *The Edwin Smith Surgical Papyrus.* Published in facsimile and hieroglyphic transliteration with translation and commentary in two volumes. Chicago, U. of Chicago, 1930.
2. Gordon, B. L.: *Medicine Throughout Antiquity.* Philadelphia, Davis, 1949.
3. Hurry, J. B.: *Imhotep, The Vizier and Physician of King Zoser and Afterwards the Egyptian God of Medicine.* Humphrey Milford, Oxford U. P., 1926.
4. Murray, M. A.: *Egypt.* Philosophical Library, New York, 1949.
5. Sigerist, H. E.: *A History of Medicine, Vol. I, Primitive and Ar-*

*chaic Medicine*. New York, Oxford U. P., 1951.

VI *Greek, Roman and Arabic Medicine*

1. Adams, F.: *The Genuine Works of Hippocrates*. Baltimore, Williams and Wilkins, 1939.
2. Chadwick, J., and Mann, W. N.: *The Medical Works of Hippocrates*. Oxford, Blackwell Scientific Publications, 1950.
3. Elgood, C.: *A Medical History of Persia and the Eastern Caliphate*. Cambridge, Cambridge U. P., 1951.
4. Green, R. M.: *Galen's Hygiene*. Springfield, Ill., Thomas, 1951.
5. Peterson, W. F.: *Hippocratic Wisdom*. Springfield, Ill., Thomas, 1946.
6. Singer, C.: *Galen On Anatomical Procedures*. New York, Oxford U. P., 1956.
7. Temkin, O.: *Soranus' Gynecology*. Baltimore, Johns Hopkins, 1956.

VII *Medieval and Renaissance Medicine*

1. Ball, J. M.: *Andreas Vesalius, The Reformer of Anatomy*. St. Louis, Medical Science Press, 1910.
2. Belt, E.: *Leonardo The Anatomist*. Lawrence, Kansas, U. of Kans., 1955.
3. Campbell, E., and Colton, J.: *The Surgery of Theodoric*. New York, Appleton, 1955.
4. Hamby, W. B.: *The Case Reports and Autopsy Reports of Ambroise Paré*. Springfield, Ill., Thomas, 1960.
5. Lambert, S. W.; Wiegard, W., and Ivins Jr., W. M.: *Three Vesalian Essays*. New York, Macmillan, 1952.
6. Lind, L. R.; Asling, C. W., and Clendening, L.: *The Epitome of Andreas Vesalius*. New York, Macmillan, 1949.
7. Pachter, H. M.: *Paracelsus*. New York, Henry Schuman, 1952.
8. Keynes, G.: *The Apologie and Treatise of Ambroise Paré Containing the Voyages made into Divers Places*. London, Falcon Educational Books, 1951.
9. Saunders, J. B. de C., and O'Malley, C. D.: *The Illustrations From the Works of Andreas Vesalius of Brussels*. Cleveland and New York, World Book Publishing Co., 1950.
10. Singer, C.: *The Hidden Causes of Disease by Antonio Benivieni*. Springfield, Ill., Thomas, 1954.

VIII *Seventeenth and Eighteenth Century Medicine*

1. Alexander, B.: *The Seats and Causes of Diseases Investigated by Anatomy*, 3 vols., Trans. from the Latin of John Baptist Morgagni. New York, Hafner, 1960.
2. Cohen, I. B.: *Benjamin Franklin, Some Account of the Pennsylvania Hospital*. Baltimore, Johns Hopkins Press, 1954.
3. Feindel, W.: *Thomas Willis, The Anatomy of the Brain and Nerves*, 2 vols. Montreal, McGill Univ., 1965.
4. Franklin, K. J.: *De Motu Cordis by William Harvey*. Springfield, Ill., Thomas, 1957.
5. Franklin, K. J.: *De Venarum Ostiolis 1603 of Hieronymus Fabricius of Aquapendente*. Springfield, Ill., Thomas, 1933.
6. Gordon, M. B.: *Aesculapius Comes to the Colonies*. Ventnor, N. J., Ventnor, 1949.
7. Leake, C. D.: *Anatomical Studies on the Motion of the Heart and Blood by William Harvey, M.D.*, Springfield, Ill., Thomas, 1928.

IX *Nineteenth and Twentieth Century Medicine*


A. *Nursing*

1. AUSTIN, ANNE L.: *History of Nursing Source Book.* New York, Putnam, 1957.
2. BAUMAN, SISTER MARY BEATA: *A Way of Mercy, Catherine McAuley's Contribution to Nursing.* New York, Vantage, 1958.
3. DOLAN, JOSEPHINE A.: *Goodnow's History of Nursing, 10th Ed.* London, Saunders, 1958, p. 422.
4. SELLEW, GLADYS, and EBEL, SISTER M.: *Ethelreda: A History of Nursing.* St. Louis, Mosby, 1955.

B. *Medical*

1. BAILEY, PEARCE: *J.-M. Charcot, 1825–1893, His Life—His Work by Georges Guillain, M.D.* New York, Hoeber Medical Div., 1959.
2. COPE, Z.: *The History of the Royal College of Surgeons of England.* London, Anthony Blond, 1959.
3. CUSHING, H.: *The Medical Career.* Boston, Little, 1940.
4. CUSHING, H.: *The Life of Sir William Osler.* New York, Oxford U. P.: 1946.
5. DAVIS, L.: *The Fellowship of Surgeons, A History of the American College of Surgeons.* Springfield, Ill., Thomas, 1960.
6. FLEXNER, S. and FLEXNER, J. H.: *William Henry Welch and the Heroic Age of American Medicine.* New York, Viking, 1941.
7. FULTON, J. F.: *Harvey Cushing, A Biography.* Springfield, Ill., Thomas, 1946.
8. GLASSER, O.: *Dr. W. C. Roëntgen.* Springfield, Ill., Thomas, 1945.
9. GODLEE, J. G.: *Lord Lister.* London, Macmillan, 1918.
10. GREENE, H. E., HENDERSON, L. J. and COHEN, I. B.: *An Introduction to the Study of Experimental Medicine by Claude Bernard.* Dover, New York, 1957.
11. GREENHILL, W. A.: *Sir Thomas Browne's Religio Medici.* London, Macmillan, 1950.
12. HURWITZ, A. and DEGENSHEIN, G. A.: *Milestones in Modern Surgery.* New York, Harper, 1958.
13. MARTÍ-IBÁÑEZ, FÉLIX (Ed.): *History of American Medicine, A Symposium.* New York, M.D. Pub., 1958.
14. MILLIS, JOHN S.: *The Graduate Education of Physicians.* Chicago, American Medical Association, 1966.
15. OSLER, W.: *Aequanimitas, With other Addresses to the Medical Students, Nurses and Practitioners of Medicine.* Philadelphia, Blakiston, 1904.
16. SCHÜCK, H.; SOHLMAN, R.; ÖSTERLING, A.; LILJESTRAND, G.; WESTGREN, A.; SIEGBAHM, M.; SCHON, A., and STÄHLE, N. K.: *Nobel, The Man and His Prizes,* Amsterdam, Elsevier Publishing Co., 1962.
17. SIGERSON, G.: *Lectures on The Diseases of the Nervous System by J.-M. Charcot.* New York, Hafner, 1962.
18. The National Health Education Committee, Inc.: *Facts on the Major Killing and Crippling Diseases in the United States Today,* 1966 Edition. 866 United Nations Plaza, New York, N.Y., 10017.
19. THORWALD, JÜRGEN: *The Century of the Surgeon.* New York, Pantheon, 1957.
20. ZIMMERMAN, L. M. and VEITH, ILZA: *Great Ideas in the History of Surgery.* Baltimore, Williams and Wilkins, 1961.

*What's past is prologue.* William Shakespeare

*We are tied down, all our days, and for the greater part of our days, to the commonplace. That is where contact with great thinkers, great literature, helps. In their company we are still in the ordinary world, but it is the ordinary world transfigured and seen through eyes of wisdom and genius. And some of their vision becomes our own.*—SIR RICHARD LIVINGSTONE

# Index of Names and Subjects

## I NAMES

## II SUBJECTS